PHARMACOLOGY

CLASSIFICATION
&
DOSES
(Dosage of all the drugs at the end of the book)

SECOND EDITION

BY

Major (Retd)
DR. SAIF-UD-DIN SAIF
M.B;B.S, M.P.H, RMP, RHMP
Professor of Community Medicine

(All rights of publication and translation of this book are reserved with the writer)

First Edition: *April 2006*
Second Edition: *April 2020*

Author: *Maj (Retd)*
DR. SAIF-UD-DIN SAIF
M.B;B.S, M.P.H, RMP, RHMP
Teaching experience of 24 years at M.B.B.S and post graduate level in various medical colleges of Pakistan.
Cell Phone / Whatsapp: +92321-5827435
Email: drsaif1919@gmail.com

Bibliography

1. *Bertram G. Katzung*, Ninth Edition: Basic and Clinical Pharmacology, California, San Francisco
2. Ronald H. Girdwood: *Dilling Clinical Pharmacology* 10th Edition
3. Alfred Goodman Gilman, Louis S. Goodman, Alfred Gilman: *Goodman and Gilman's The Pharmacological Basis of Therapeutic*, Virginia.
4. Richard D Howland, Mary J. Mycek: *Lippincott's Illustrated Reviews*, New Jersy.

Preface

This book is designed to provide a complete, comprehensive, current and quick information about the various drug classes and their doses. The classifications of various drug groups have been given according to the following characreristics.

    a. Chemical Composition
    b. Mechanism of Action
    c. Duration of Action
    d. Site of Action in the human body
    e. Therapeutic Classification
    f. Solubility of the drugs
    g. Selectivity of the drugs
    h. Agonistic Action
    i. Antagonistic Action
    j. Mode of Usage: Systemic or Topical

The index of Major Drug Groups is given on page 5 to 8 and a detailed index with dosage is given at the end of the book. The abbreviations used are as under.

IM	Intramuscular
IV	Intravenous
PR	Per rectum
SC	Subcutaneous
SL	Sublingual
Od	Once daily
bid	Twice daily
tid	Three times a day
qid	Four times a day

mg	Milligram
g	Gram
mcg or µgm	Microgram
sq. m	Body surface area in square meter
ID	Intradermal
IU	International unit

This book has been especially designed and compiled for the Undergraduate Medical Students, the Internee Officers, the Postgraduate Students and the Pharmacy Students.

I am thankful to Almighty Allah for giving me the faculties to conceive the idea and strength and resources to compile this noble task.

I dedicate this work to my wife, my parents and my honourable teachers. I am thankful to my worthy colleagues for their help, cooperation and encouragement.

Suggestions and comments are always welcome.

Major (Retd)
Professor DR. SAIF-UD-DIN SAIF
M.B;B.S, M.P.H, RMP, RHMP.
Specialist Community Medicine
Rawalpindi, Pakistan

24-April-2020

MAJOR DRUG GROUPS

I. AUTONOMIC DRUGS   9
   Cholinergic Drugs (Parasympathomimetics)
   Anticholinesterases
   Cholinesterase Inhibitors
   Anticholinergic Drugs
   Cholinergic Blocking Drugs
   Central Nervous System Stimulants
   Adrenoceptor Activating & other Sympathomimetc Drugs
   Sympathomimetics (α & β blockers)
   Classification of α Blockers
   Classification of β Blockers
   Adrenal Steroid Inhibitors

II. CARDIOVASCULAR-RENAL DRUGS   21
   Anti-Hypertensive Drugs
   Vasodilators
   Vasoconstrictors
   Anti-Anginal Drugs
   Organic Nitrites and Nitrates
   Drugs used in Heart Failure
   Anti-Arrhythmic Drugs
   Diuretics

**III. DRUGS WITH IMPORTANT ACTION ON
      SMOOTH MUSCLES**   37
   Antihistamines, Serotonin, & Ergot Alkaloids
   H-1 Receptor Blockers
   Kinins
   Vasoactive Peptide, Substance P
   Eicosanoids (Prostaglandins,Thromboxanes,Leukotrienes)
   Bronchial Asthma
   Bronchodilators

IV. CENTRAL NERVOUS SYSTEM   44
Sedatives-Hypnotics
Acute Alcohol Withdrawal Syndrome
Drugs for Prevention of Alcohol Abuse
Treatment of Acute Methanol or Ethylene Glycol Poisoning
Anti-Epileptic/Anti-seizure Drugs
General Anesthetics
Local Anesthetics
Skeletal Muscle Relaxants
Parkinsonism and other Movement Disorders
Psychotropic Drugs
Anti-Psychotic Drugs
Anti-Anxiety Drugs
Benzodiazepines
Anti-Depressants
Psycho-mimetic Drugs
Mood Stabilizers
Analgesics-Narcotic
Central Nervous System Depressants
Drugs of Abuse

V. DISEASES OF BLOOD, INFLAMMATION & GOUT   63
Anaemias, Haemopoietic growth factors
Haemostatics (Coagulants)
Anti-Coagulants
Fibrinolytic (Thrombolytic Drugs)
Anti-Platelet Drugs
Anti-Lipidemic Drugs
Non-Steroidal Anti-Inflammatory Drugs
Disease Modifying Anti-Rheumatic Drugs
Drugs used in Gout

VI. ENDOCRINE DRUGS   71
Hypothalamic and Anterior/Posterior Pituitary Hormones
Hyperthyroidism (Anti-thyroid Drugs)
Thyroid Storm (thyroid crisis)

Non-toxic Goiter
Hypothyroidism (Thyroid Agents)
Adrenocoticosteroids
Adrenocoticosteroids Antagonists
Glucocorticoids
Gonadal Hormones and Inhibitors
Androgens and Anabolic Steroids
Pancreatic Hormones and Anti-Diabetic Drugs
Bone Mineral Homeostasis

VII. CHEMOTHERAPEUTIC DRUGS 81
Antibiotics
Anti-Viral Agents
Disinfectants, Antiseptics and Sterilants
Anti-Protozoal Drugs (malaria, amoebiasis, trichomoniasis, giardiasis, leishmaniasis)
Anti-Fungal Drugs
Anthelmitic Drugs
Cancer Chemotherapy
Tuberculosis
Immunopharmacology/Immunomodulants
Agents for Active Immunization in USA
Agents for Passive Immunization in USA

VIII. TOXICOLOGY 108
Heavy Metal Intoxication & Chelators
Poisons and their Antidotes

IX. SPECIAL TOPICS 109
Anti-Leprosy Drugs
Drugs used in Venereal Diseases
Vaccines and Sera/Immunoglobulins
Anti-Diarrhoeal Drugs
Irritable Bowel Syndrome (IBS)
Inflammatory Bowel Diseases (IBD)
Varices Haemorrahge
Digestants
Appetite suppressants

Anti-Emetics /Emetics
Bitters
Anti-Tussives
Carbonic Anhydrase Inhibitors
Digestive Enzymes
Expectorant/Mucolytics
Respiratory Stimulants
Drugs used in Gall bladder Diseases
Gallstones Dissolving Agents
Open Angle Glaucoma

X. GASTROINTESTINAL TRACT 119
Anti-Inflammatory Drugs for GIT Diseases
Drugs used in Peptic ulcer/H. pylori
Sialogogues/Anti-Sialogogues
Motility Disorders & Selected Anti-Emetics
Purgatives/Laxatives

XI. MISCELLANEOUS 126
Special Aspects of Peri-natal & Paediatric Pharmacology
Drugs used during Lactation & their Effects on Nursing Infant
Erectile Dysfunction (ED)
Osteoporosis
Obesity
Dermatological Pharmacology
Drugs that Enhance Drug Metabolism
Drugs that Inhibit Drug Metabolism

AUTONOMIC DRUGS

CHOLINERGIC DRUGS
(Parasympathomimetics)

A. Directly Acting
B. Indirectly Acting
A. **DIRECTLY ACTING CHOLINERGIC DRUGS**
   I. **CHOLINE ESTERS**
      1. Acetylcholine
      2. Methacholine chloride
      3. Carbachol chloride
      4. Bethanechol chloride
   II. **CHOLINOMIMETIC NATURAL ALKALOIDS**
      1. **Mainly Muscarinic Agonists**
         a. **Natural Alkaloids**
            1. Muscarine
            2. Pilocarpine
            3. Arecholine
         b. **Synthetic Alkaloid**
            Oxotramorine
      2. **Mainly Nicotinic Agonists**
         a. **Natural Alkaloids**
            1. Nicotine
            2. Lobeline
         b. **Synthetic Alkaloids**
            Dimethylphenylpiperazinium (DMPP)
      3. **Miscellaneous**
         Cevimeline (for dry mouth in Sjogren syndrome)
B. **INDIRECTLY ACTING CHOLINERGIC DRUGS**
(Anti-Cholinesterases, Cholinesterase Inhibitors)

1. **Alcohols** bearing a quaternary ammonium group:
    1. Edrophonium   2. Ambenonium

2. Carbamic Acid Esters of Alcohols bearing quaternary or tertiary ammonium group:
   Carbamates: Neostigmine
3. Organic Derivatives of Phosphoric Acid (Organophosphates)
   Echothiophate

ANTICHOLINESTERASES

I. REVERSIBLE ANTICHOLINESTERASES

1. CARBAMATES
   Tertiary Amines
      Physostigmine, eserine
   Quaternary Ammonium Compounds
      1. Neostigmine
      2. Pyridostigmine
      3. Distigmine
      4. Ambenonium
      5. Demecarium
2. SIMPLE ALCOHOLS bearing a quaternary ammonium group: Edrophonium
3. MISCELLANEOUS (mainly used in Alzheimer's disease)
      1. Tacrine
      2. Donepezil
      3. Galantamine
      4. Rivastigmine

II. IRREVERSIBLE ANTICHOLINESTERASES
   (Organophosphorus Compounds)
   1. Therapeutically useful: Echothiophate
   2. War Gases: Sarin, Tuban, Soman
   3. Insecticides: Parathion, Malathion

CHOLINESTRERASE INHIBITORS
(Therapeutic Uses and Duration of Action)

	Uses	Duration of action
Alcohols Edrophoniun	Myesthenia gravis, ileus, arrhythmia	5-15 minutes
Carbamates and related agents		
Neostigmine	Myesthenia gravis, ileus	0.5-2 hours
Pyridostigmine	Myesthenia gravis	3-6 hours
Physostigmine	Glaucoma	0.5-2 hours
Ambenonium	Myesthenia gravis	4-8 hours
Demacarium	Glaucoma	4-6 hours
Organophosphates		
Echothiophate	Glaucoma	10 hours

ANTICHOLINERGIC DRUGS
(Therapeutic Classification)

1. **ANTI-SPASMODIC (Spasmolytics)**
   1. Atropine sulphate
   2. Hyoscine Hydrobromide
   3. Clidinium
   4. Propantheline
   5. Dicyclomine
2. **DRUGS FOR PEPTIC ULCER**
   1. Pirenzepine
   2. Telenzepine
3. **DRUGS FOR URINARY INCONTINENCE**
   1. Oxybutynin
   2. Propiverine
   3. Tolterodine (M 3 selective blocker)
4. **MOTION SICKNESS**
   Hyoscine
5. **MYDRIATRICS & CYCLOPLEGICS**
   1. Atropine sulphate
   2. Hyoscine, belladonna alkaloids, extract or tincture

      3. Homatropine
      4. Cyclopentolate
      5. Tropicamide
      6. Eucatropine
6. **DRUGS FOR BRONCHIAL ASTHMA**
    1. Ipratropium
    2. Tiotropium
7. **DRUGS FOR PARKINSONISM**
    1. Benztropine   2. Benzhexol
    3. Biperidine   4. Procyclidine

CHOLINERGIC BLOCKING DRUGS
(Antimuscarinic or Parasympatholytic Drugs)
(Chemical Classification)

I. **Natural Belladonna Alkaloids, extract or tincture**
    1. Atropine
    2. Hyoscine
    3. l-hyoscyamine

II. **Semisynthetic and Synthetic Substitutes of Belladonna Alkaloids (Atropine-like Drugs)**
    a. **Tertiary-Amine Compounds**
        1. Dicyclomine HCl
        2. Oxyphencyclimine HCl
        3. Thiphenamil HCl
        4. Methixene HCl
        5. Piperidolate HCl
        6. Homatropine Hydrobromide
        7. Cyclopentolate HCl
        8. Eucatropine HCl
        9. Tropicamide
    b. **Quaternary Ammonium Derivatives**
        1. Atropine Methobromide
        2. Atropine Methonitrate
        3. Hyoscine Butylbromide
        4. Hyoscine Methobromide

5. Clidinium
6. Cyclopentolate

CENTRAL NERVOUS SYSTEM STIMULANTS

1. **CEREBRAL STIMULANTS**
    i. **Xanthines**: Caffeine, Theophylline, Theobromine
    ii. **Sympathomimetics**: Ephedrine, Amphetamine
    iii. **Parasympatholytics**: Atropine
    iv. **Local anaesthetics**: Coacine
2. **BRAIN STEM STIMULANTS(Analeptics, Restoratives)**
    Nikethamide, Picrotoxin, Bemergide, Ethamivan, Doxapram
3. **SPINAL CORD STIMULANTS**
    i. Nux vomica
    ii. Morphine

ADRENOCEPTOR-ACTIVATING AND OTHER SYMPATHOMIMETIC DRUGS

SYMPATHOMIMETICS
(According to Receptors)

1. **DRUGS ACTING ON α & β RECEPTORS**
    1. Epinephrine
    2. Norepinephrine (Noradrenaline)
    3. Ephedrine
    4. Amphetamine & Congeners
    5. Metaraminol
    6. Mephentermine
2. **DRUGS ACTING ON β RECEPTOR ($\beta_1 + \beta_2$)**
    Isoprenaline or Isoproterenol
3. **DRUGS ACTING ON β_1 RECEPTOR**
    (Selective β_1 Agonists)
    1. Prenalterol   2. Dobutamine

4. **DRUGS ACTING ON β_2 RECEPTOR**
   (Selective β_2 Agonists)
   1. Terbutaline
   2. Salmeterol
   3. Albuterol
   4. Tulbuterol
   5. Rimiterol
   6. Metaproterenol
   7. Fenoterol
   8. Ritodrine
   9. Pirbuterol

5. **DRUGS ACTING ON α RECEPTOR (α_1, α_2)**
   1. Metaraminol
   2. Mephentermine
   3. Xylometazoline
   4. Oxymetazoline
   5. Naphazoline

6. **DRUGS ACTING ON α_1 RECEPTOR**
   (α_1 AGONIST)
   1. Methoxamine
   2. Phenylephrine
   3. Midodrine

7. **DRUGS ACTING ON α_2 RECEPTOR**
   (SELECTIVE α_2 AGONIST)
   1. Methyldopa
   2. Clonidine
   3. Primonidine
   4. Apraclonidine
   5. Guanfacine
   6. Guanabenz
   7. Dexmedetomidine (for sedation of the critically ill)
   8. Tizanidine

8. **Dopamine agonists**
   1. Dopamine
   2. Fenoldapam

SYMPATHOMIMETICS
(According to Mode of Action)

A. DIRECTLY ACTING SYMPATHOMIMETICS
1. Adrenaline
2. Noradrenaline
3. Salmetrol
4. Terbutaline
5. Mephentermine
6. Dopamine
7. Clonidine

B. INDIRECTLY ACTING SYMPATHOMIMETICS
1. Tyramine
2. Ephedrine
3. Pseudoephedrine
4. Amphetamine
5. Phenylmetrazine (anorexiants)
6. Methylphenidate (Attention defecit hyperactivity syndrome)
7. Pemoline

SYMPATHOMIMETICS
(Chemical Classification)

A. Catecholamines
Natural
1. Adrenaline
2. Noradrenaline
3. Dopamine

Synthetic
1. Isoprenaline
2. Dobutamine
3. Rimiterol
4. Isoetharine
5. Hexoprenaline

B. Non-Catecholamines
1. Ephedrine
2. Pseudoephedrine
3. Amphetamine
4. Dexamphetamine
5. Methylamphetamine
6. Salbutamol
7. Terbutaline
8. Methoxamine

SYMPATHOMIMETICS
(Therapeutic Classification)

I. **Used in the Treatment of Bronchial Asthma**
1. Salbutamol
2. Orciprenaline
3. Pseudoephedrine
4. Isoetharine
5. Rimiterol
6. Procarterol
7. Terbutaline
8. Ephedrine
9. Adrenaline
10. Methoxyphenamine
11. Phenylpropranolamine

II. **Used in the Treatment of Nasal Congsetion**
1. Ephedrine
2. Pseudoephedrine
3. Phenylephrine
4. Phenylpropranolamine
5. Methoxamine
6. Naphazoline
7. Mephentermine
8. Propylhexidrine
9. Tetrahydrozoline
10. Oxymetazoline
11. Xylometazoline

III. **Used in the Treatment of Hypotension**
1. Metaraminol
2. Dopamine
3. Phenylephrine
4. Phenylpropanolamine
5. Adrenaline(acute anaphylaxis)
6. Methoxamine
7. Ephedrine
8. Noradrenaline
9. Mephentermine
10. Oxedrine

IV. **Used in the Treatment of Heart Block**
1. Adrenaline
2. Ephedrine
3. Isoprenaline

V. **Used in Prevention of Premature Labour**
1. Salbutamol
2. Terbutaline
3. Ritodrine
4. Isoxsuprine
5. Fenoterol

VI. **Used as Vasodilators (in peripheral vascular disease)**

    1. Isoxsuprine   2. Nyldrin
VII. **Used as CNS Stimulants**
    1. Amphetamine   3. Dexamphetamine
    2. Methamphetamine
VIII. **Used as Anorexic Agents (in obesity)**
    1. Phenmetrazine   3. Phenfluramine
    2. Amphetamine   4. Dexamphetamine
IX. **Used as Mydriatics**
    1. Phenylephrine   3. Ephedrine
    2. Adrenaline

CLASSIFICATION OF α BLOCKERS
(According to Receptor Selectivity)

1. **NON-SELECTIVE ALPHA BLOCKERS (Both α_1 & α_2)**
   1. Phentolamine
   2. Tolazoline
2. **SELECTIVE α_1 BLOCKERS (Postsynaptic)**
   1. Prazosin
   2. Terazosin
   3. Doxazosin
   4. Tamsulosin (α_{1A} blocker)
   5. Alfuzosin
   6. Indoramin
3. **PREDOMINANTLY α_1 (Post-Synaptic) BLOCKERS**
   1. Phenoxybenzamine (Irreversible)
   2. Urapidil

4. **SELECTIVE α_2 BLOCKERS (Post-synaptic)**
       Yohimbine
5. **BOTH α_1 & β BLOCKERS**
   1. Labetalol
   2. Carvedilol
6. **Other Drugs Possessing α blockig Activity**
   1. Phenothiazines   3. Trazodone
   2. Butyrophnones   4. Pizotifen

α BLOCKERS
(Chemical Classification)

A. **QUINAZOLINE DERIVATIVES**
   1. Prazosin
   2. Trimazosin
B. **ERGOT ALKALOIDS**
   1. Ergotoxine (ergocornine, ergocriptine, ergocristine)
   2. Ergotamine
   3. Dihydroergotoxine
   4. Dihydroergotamine
A. **HALOALKYLAMINES**
   1. Phenoxybenzamine
   2. Dibenamine
D. **BENZYL IMIDAZOLINE DERIVATIVES**
   1. Phentolamine
   2. Tolazoline
E. **PHENOTHIAZINES & BUTYROPHENONES**
   1. Chlorpromazine
   2. Haloperidol
F. **INDOLE ALKYLAMINE DERIVATIVES**
   Yohimbine
G. **MISCELLANEOUS**
   1. Prazocin
   2. Indoramin
   3. Labetolol (Both α and β receptor blocking agents)

α BLOCKERS
(Based on Duration of Action)

REVERSIBLE
1. Phentolamine
2. Tolazoline
3. Prazocin

IRREVERSIBLE: Phenoxybenzamine dibenamine

β-BLOCKERS
(According to Selectivity)

A. NON-SELECTIVE (β$_1$, β$_2$) BLOCKERS
1. Pure Blockers
    1. Sotalol
    2. Timolol (ophthalmic)
    3. Nadolol
    4. Levobunolol
    5. Metoprolol
2. With Membrane Stabilizing Activity (MSA)
    Propanolol
3. With Intrinsic Sympathetic Activity (ISA)
    1. Penbutolol
    2. Carteolol (Eye drops)
4. With ISA & MSA
    1. Oxprenolol
    2. Alprenolol
    3. Pindolol

B. CARDIOSELECTIVE (β1) BLOCKERES
1. Pure Blockers
    1. Atenolol   3. Bisoprolol
    2. Esmolol   4. Nebivolol (Ophthalmic drops)
2. With MSA
    1. Metoprolol   3. Tolamolol
    2. Betaxolol
3. With ISA
    Practalol
4. With ISA & MSA
    Acebutalol

C. BOTH α$_1$ & β BLOCKERS
1. Labetalol   2. Carvedilol
3. Medroxalol   4. Bucinodolol

D. β$_1$ BLOCKER WITH PARTIAL β$_2$ AGONIST ACTIVITY
   Celiprolol

β-BLOCKERS
(According to Solubility)

I. **LIPID SOLUBLE**
    1. Propranolol
    2. Pindolol
    3. Timolol
    4. Metoprolol

II. **WATER SOLUBLE**
    1. Nadolol
    2. Atenolol

β-BLOCKERS
(According to Duration of Action)

I. **ULTRA SHORT ACTING**
    Esmolol: $t\ \frac{1}{2}$ 10min

II. **INTERMEDIATE ACTING**

1. Propranolol	3-5 hours
2. Domolol	3-5 hours
3. Pindolol	3-4 hours
4. Metoprolol	3-4 hours

III. **LONG ACTING**

1. Nadolol	10-20 hours
2. Atenolol	05-08 hours
3. Bisoprolol	09-12 hours
4. Sotalol	12 hours
5. Betaxolol	14-22 hours

ADRENAL STEROID INHIBITORS

    1. Aminoglutethimide
    2. Ketaconazole
    3. Mitotane

CARDIOVASCULAR-RENAL DRUGS

ANTI-HYPERTENSIVE DRUGS

I. **DIURETICS**
   (a) **Thiazides**
      1. Bendrofluazide
      2. Chlorthalidone
      3. Polythiazide
      4. Hydrochlorothiazide
      5. Cyclopenthiazide
   (b) **Loop Diuretics**
      1. Furosemide
      2. Ethacrynic acid
      3. Bumetanide

II. **SYMPATHOLYTIC DRUGS (Sympathoplegics)**
   1. **Centrally Acting Drugs**
      1. α Methyldopa
      2. Clonidine
      3. Guanabenz
      4. Guanfacine
   2. **β-Adrenergic Receptor Antagonists**

1. Propranolol	7. Metoprolol
2. Acebutalol	8. Betaxolol
3. Bisoprolol	9. Carteolol
4. Carvedilol	10. Nadolol
5. Penbutolol	11. Pindolol
6. Timolol	

   3. **α-Adrenergic Receptor Antagonists**
      1. Prazosin   2. Phenoxybenzamine
   4. **Alpha & Beta Antagonists**
      Labetalol

5. **Adrenergic Neuron Blockers**
   1. Guanethidine
   2. Reserpine
   3. Guanadrel
6. **Ganglion Blocking Agents**
   Trimetaphan

III. **CALCIUM CHANNEL BLOCKERS**
   1. **Dihydropyridines**
      1. Nifedipine
      2. Nicardipine
      3. Nimodipine
      4. Amlodipine
      5. Nisoldipine
      6. Nitrendipine
      7. Felodipine
      8. Isradipine
   2. **Phenylalkylamines**
      1. Verapamil
      2. Gallopamil
   3. **Piperazines**
      1. Flunarizine
      2. Trimetazidine
      3. Ranolazine
   4. **Miscellaneous**
      1. Diltiazem
      2. Bepridine

IV. **VASODILATORS**
   1. **Arteriolar Vasodilators**
      1. Hydralazine
      2. Minoxidil
      3. Diazoxide
      4. Fenoldopam
   2. **Arteriolar and Venular Vasodilators**
      1. Sodium Nitroprusside
      2. Prazocin

V. **ANGIOTENSIN-CONVERTING ENZYME INIBITORS**
   (a) **Drugs Inhibiting Release of Renin**
      Propranolol and other β-Blockers
   (b) **Drugs Inhibitng Angiotensin Converting Enzyme (ACE-Inhibitors)**

1. Captopril
2. Cilazapril
3. Quinapril
4. Perindopril
5. Losartan
6. Enalapril
7. Lisinopril
8. Fosinopril
9. Remipril
10. Candesartan

(c) Drugs Blocking Renin at Receptor
Saralasin

VI. ADRENERGIC NEURONE BLOCKERS
(Anti-adrenergic Drugs)

1. Drugs that Prevent Release of Noradrenaline
1. Guanathidine
2. Debrisoquine
3. Guanadrel
4. Bethanidine
5. Guanoxan
6. Bretylium

2. Drugs that Inhibit Storage of Noradrenaline
1. Reserpine
2. Syrosingopine
3. Alseroxylon
4. Deserpidine
5. Rescinnamine

3. Drugs that Interfere with Synthesis of Noradrenaline
1. Methyldopa
2. Metyrosine

VII. GANGLION BLOCKING DRUGS
1. Quaternary Ammonium Compounds
1. Hexamethonium
2. Pentamethonium
3. Pentolinium tartrate

2. Secondary Amines: Mecamylamine
3. Tertiary Amines: Pempidine
4. Sulphonium Compounds: Trimetaphan

VIII. INHIBITORS OF ANGIOTENSIN
Angiotensin-Converting Enzyme (ACE) Inhibitors
1. Captoril
2. Fosinopril
3. Benazepril
4. Quinapril
7. Enalapril
8. Lisinopril
9. Trandolapril
10. Moexipril

    5. Ramipril   11. Imidapril
    6. Perindopril

IX. ANGIOTENSIN RECEPTOR BLOCKERS (ARBs) (Angiotensin Type-I Blockers)
1. Losartan
2. Candesartan
3. Valsartan
4. Eprosartan
5. Irbesartan
6. Telmisartan
7. Saralasin

X. Tyrosine Hydroxylase Inhibitors: Metyrosine
XI. Monoamine Oxidase Inhibitors: Pargyline
XII. Drugs Acting on Afferent Nerve Endings
    Veratrum Alkaloids: Protoveratrine A & B

VASODILATORS
(Therapeutic Classification)

I. Vasodilators for Angina Pectoris
1. Glyceryl trinitrate
2. Isosorbide dinitrate

II. Vasodilators for Heart Failure
  a. Venodilators (decrease preload by increasing venous capacitance)
    1. Glyceryl trinitrate
    2. Isosorbide dinitrate
  b. Aretriolar Dilators (reduce systemic arteriolar resistance and decrease afterload)
    1. Hydralazine
    2. Captopril
    3. Enalapril
  c. Mixed Venous and Arteriolar Dilators
    1. Sodium nitroprusside   2. Prazocin

III. Vasodilators for Hypertension
    1. Hydralazine   4. Diazoxide

    2. Minoxidil
    3. Prazocin
VI. Peripheral Vasodilators
    1. Thymoxamine
    2. Cinnarizine
    3. Cyclandelate
    4. Nicotinic acid
    5. Nicotinyl tartrate
V. Cerebral Vasodilators
    1. Co-dergocrine mesylate
    2. Naftidrofuryl

    5. Sodium nitroprusside
    6. Thiazides

    6. Isoxsuprine
    7. Oxypentifylline
    8. Inositol nicotinate
    9. Nicofuranose
    10. Naftidrofuryl

    3. Cyclandelate
    4. Isoxsuprine

VASODILTORS
(Site of Action)

I. ACTING ON VASCULAR SMOOTH MUSCLES

  a. Nitrites and Nitrates
    1. Glyceyl trinitrate
    2. Isosorbide dinitrate
    3. Isosorbide mononitrate
    4. Pentaerythritol tetranitrate
    5. Erythritol tetranitrate
    6. Mannitol hexanitrate
    7. Amyl nitrate
  b. Benzothiadiazides
    1. Thiazides
    2. Diazoxide
  c. Xanthines
    1. Aminophylline   2. Oxipentifylline
    3. Xanthinol nicotinate
  d. Derivatives of Nicotinic acid
    1. Nicotinic acid
    2. Nicofuranose
    3. Nicotinyl alcohol
    4. Nicotinyl tartrate

    5. Inositol nicotinate
    6. Methyl nicotinate (for topical use)
    7. Ethyl nicotinate (for topical use)
 e. Ergot Derivatives: Co-Dergocrine Mesylate
 f. Miscellaneous
    1. Hydralazine   2. Minoxidil
    3. Sodium nitroprusside 4. Bamethan sulphate?
    5. Cyclandelate   6. Kallidinogenase
    7. Naftidrofuryl oxalate 8. Papaverine

II. ACTING ON AUTONOMIC NERVOUS SYSTEM
 a. Alpha Adrenergic Receptor Blocking Agents
    1. Prazocin
    2. Terazocin
    3. Phenoxybenzamine
    4. Thymoxamine
    5. Phentolamine (it has direct action also)
    6. Tolazoline (it has direct action also)
 b. Stimulant of Beta-Adrenergic Receptors
   (Mainly the blood vessels of skeletal muscles)
    1. Isoxuprine
    2. Salbutamol
    3. Isoprenaline
    4. Adrenaline
    5. Buphenine HCl (for Meniere's disease and the disorders of internal ear)
 c. Stimulant of Pripheral Dopaminergic Receptors
   Dopamine (in renal, mesenteric, coronary and intracerebral vessels)
 d. Anticholinergics: Atropine (in large dose)

III. CALCIUM CHANNEL BLOCKERS
    1. Nifedipine   2. Nicardipine
    3. Amlodipine   4. Isradipine
    5. Felodipine   6. Nimodipine
    7. Diltiazim   8. Lidoflazine
    9. Prenylamine lactate 10. Perhexilline maleate

IV. ANGIOTENSIN CONVERTING ENZYME INHIBITORS

1. Captopril
2. Enalapril
3. Cilazapril
4. Fosinopril
5. Lisinopril
V. HISTAMINE AND ANTIHISTAMINES
1. Histamine
2. Cinnarizine
VI. DEPRESSANTS OF VASOMOTOR CENTRE
1. Alcohol
2. Morphine (partly through release of histamine)
VII. LOCAL ANAESTHETICS: All local anaesthetics except cocaine

VASOCONSTRICTORS

I. CENTRALLY ACTING (Stimulants of Vasomotor Center)
a. Drugs Acting Directly
i. *Analeptics*
1. Nikethamide
2. Doxapram
3. Ethamivan
4. Penetrazol
5. Bemergide
6. Amiphenazole
7. Picrotoxin

ii. *Xanthines*
1. Caffeine   2. Theophylline
3. Aminophylline

b. Drugs Acting Reflexly (Mild Peripheral Irritants)
1. Ammonium inhalation
2. Aromatic spirit of ammonia
3. Camphor, subcutaneously

II. PERIPHERALLY ACTING VASOCONSTRICTORS
a. Stimulants of Alpha-Adrenergic Receptors
(Sympathomimetics)

1. Adrenaline
2. Noradrenaline
3. Phenylephrine
4. Methoxamine
5. Metaraminol
6. Mephentermine
7. Ephedrine
8. Amphetamines

b. Stimulants of Sympathetic Ganglia: Nicotine

c. Partial Agonists of Alpha-Adrenergic Receptors
1. Ergotamine tartrate (used for migraine)
2. Dihydoergotamine
3. Ergometrine

d. Direct Stimulants of Vascular Smooth Muscle
1. Vasopressin (ADH)
2. Lypressin (Synthetic Lysine-Vasopressin)
3. Angiotensin
4. Xanthines (direct vasoconstriction of cerebral vessels)

e. Miscellaneous
Cocaine (partly by inhibition of reuptake of neurotransmitters by adrenergic neurones

ANTI-ANGINAL DRUGS

1. **ORGANIC NITRATES**
    (a) Rapidly Acting Drugs
    Glyceryl trinitrate (Nitroglycerin)
    Amyl nitrate
    (b) Drugs with Prolonged Action
    Isosorbide dinitrate
    Isosorbide mononitrate
    Pentaerythritol tetranitrate
    Erythrityl tetranitrate

2. β ADRENOCEPTOR BLOCKERS
   a. Propranolol
   b. Acebutalol
   c. Atenolol
   d. Metoprolol
   e. Nadolol

3. CALCIUM CHANNEL BLOCKERS
   a. **Dihydropyridine**
      1. Nitrendipine
      2. Nifedipine
      3. Amlodipine
   b. **Phenylalkylamines**
      1. Verapamil
      2. Gallopamil
   C. **Piperazines**
      1. Flunarizine
      2. Trimetazidine
      3. Ranolazine
   D. **Diltiazem**
   E. **Others**
      1. Bepridil
      2. Felodipine
      3. Isradipine
      4. Nimodipine
      5. Nisoldipine

4. MISCELLANEOUS
   Dipyridamole

5. K+ CHANNEL ACTIVATORS
   1. Cromakalim
   2. Pinacidil
   3. Nicorandil

ANTI-ANGINAL DRUGS
(Therapeutic Classification)

I. **For an Acute Attack:** Glyceryl trinitrate
II. **For Immediate Exertional Pre-exposure Prophylaxis**
    1. Glyceryl trinitrate   2. Nifedipine
III. **For Long term Prophylaxis**
   (a) **Beta Blockers:** 1. Propranolol 2. Atenolol
   (b) **Calcium Channel Blockers:** Nifedipine, Diltiazem, Verapamil
   (c) **Long Acting Nitrates:**
              Isosorbide dinitrate, Isosorbide mononitrate

ORGANIC NITRITES & NITRATES
(Duration of Action)

1. **Short Acting**
   Amyl Nitrite (inhalant) (DOA: 3-5 minutes)
   Glyceryl trinitrate (Nitroglycerine) SL:(DOA:10-30 minutes)
2. **Intermediate Acting: (DOA: 4-6 hours)**
     Isosorbide dinitrate
3. **Long Acting: (DOA: 6-8 hours)**
    1. Erythrityl tetranitrate
    2. Pentaerythritol tetranitrate
    3. Isosorbide mononitrate
    4. Glyceryl trinitrate (Trans- dermal patch)

DRUGS USED IN HEART FAILURE

A. **CARDIOTONIC DRUGS**
  1. **Cardiac Glycosides (Cardenolides)**
      1. Digoxin   4. Gitoxin
      2. Digitoxin   5. Strophanthin
      3. Ouabain   6. Gitaloxin
    Digitalis Antibody: Digoxin immune fab (ovine)
  2. **Bipyridine Derivatives**
       1. Inamrinone   2. Milrinone

3. **β1 Selective Agonists**
    1. Dobutamine
    2. Prenalterol
B. **DIURETICS**
    1. Thiazides
    2. Bendrofluazide
    3. Polythiazide
   Loop Diuretic
        Furosemide
C. **ACE INHIBITORS**
    1. Captopril
    2. Enalapril
    3. Lisinopril
D. **VASODILATORS**
    1. Hydralazine
    2. Nifedipine
    3. Prazosin
    4. Nitroglycerine
E. **BETA BLOCKERS**
    1. Carvedilol
    2. Metoprolol
    3. Bisoprolol
F. **NEW APPROACHES**
      Nestiritide (human BNP -Vasodilator)
      Omapatrilat (inhibitor of ACE, & endopipidase)

ANTI-ARRHYTHMIC DRUGS
(Cardiac Arrhythmias)

1. **SODIUM CHANNEL BLOCKING DRUGS (Class 1)**

    SUBGROUP: A
    1. Quinidine
    2. Disopyramide
    3. Encainide
    4. Procainamide
    5. Lorcainide

    SUBGROUP: B
        1. Mexiletine   3. Lignocaine
        2. Phenytoin   4. Tocainide
    SUBGROUP: C
        1. Flecainide   3. Propafenone
        2. Moricizine   4. Aprindine
2. **BETA –ADRENOCEPTOR-BLOCKING DRUGS**
    1. Acebutalol   3. Esmolol
    2. Propranolol   4. Bretylium (class III activity)
3. **ACTION POTENTIAL PROLONGING AGENTS**
    1. Amiodarone   4. Bretylium
    2. Sotalol   5. Ibutilide
    3. Dofetilide
4. **CALCIUM CHANNEL BLOCKERS**
    1. Bepridil   3. Diltiazim
    2. Verapamil
5. **MISCELLANEOUS**
    1. Adenosine
    2. Magnesium sulfate

ANTI-ARRHYTHMIC DRUGS
(Therapeutic Classification)

1. Supraventricular Arrhythmias
    1. Beta Blockers   3. Verapamil
    2. Digoxin

2. Ventricular Arrhythmias
    1. Lignocaine   3. Phenytoin
    2. Mexiletine   4. Lidocaine

3. Supraventricular and Ventricular Arrhythmias
    1. Quinidine sulfate   4. Procainamide
    2. Quinidine gluconate   5. Disopyramide
    3. Quinidine polygalacturonate   6. Aminodarone

I. DIURETICS
(Chemical Classification)

i. Mercurial Diuretics
1. Mersalyl
2. Meralluride
3. Chlormerodrin
4. Mercaptomerin
5. Merethoxylline

ii. Carbonic Anhydrase Inhibitors
1. Acetazolamide
2. Ethoxzolamide
3. Dichlorphenamide
4. Methazolamide

iii. Acidfying Salts: Ammonium chloride

iv. Thiazides (Benzothiazides, Benzothiadiazines)
1. Chlorothiazide
2. Hydrochlorothiazide
3. Hydroflumethiazide
4. Bendroflumethiazide
5. Bendroflumethiazide
6. Cyclopenthiazide
7. Polythiazide
8. Benzthiazide
9. Cyclothiazide
10. Methclothiazide
11. Trichlormethiazide

v. Thiazide-Related Compounds
Phthalimidine Derivatives
1. Chlorthalidone
2. Chlorexolone
3. Metolazone

Quinazoline derivatives: Quinethazone
Chlorobenzamide: Clopamide
Benzene Disulphonamide: Mefruside
1. Xipamide
2. Indapamide
3. Ticrynafen

vi. High-Ceiling Diuretics (Loop Diuretics)
Carboxylic Acid Derivatives

      1. Furosemide
      2. Bumetanide
      3. Piretanide
    Phenoxyacetic Acid Derivatives: Ethacrynic acid
vii. **Potassium-Sparing Diuretics**
    a. Aldosterone Antagonists
      1. Spironolactone
      2. Potassium Canrenoate
    b. Non-aldosterone Anatagonists
      1. Triamterene   2. Amiloride
viii. **Osmotic Diuretics**
      1. Mannitol   3. Urea
      2. Glycerin   4. Isosorbide
ix. **Xanthines**
      1. Aminophylline   3. Theophylline
      2. Theobromine   4. Caffeine

II. DIURETICS
(Mechanism of Action)

A. DRUGS INTERFERING WITH IONIC TRANSPORT
I. **Drugs Interfering with Ionic Transport of HCO_3^-**
    1. Acetazolamide
    2. Dichlorphenamide
    3. Methazolamide
II. **Inhibitors of Active Transport of CL^-**
  a. **THIAZIDES**
      1. Hydrochlorothiazide   5. Methylclothiazide
      2. Hydroflumethiazide   6. Chlorthalidone
      3. Chlorothiazide   7. Indapamide
      4. Benzthiazide
  b. **LOOP DIURETICS**
      1. Furosemide   5. Bumetanide
      2. Torsemide   6. Ethacrynic acid
      3. Azosemide   7. Muzolimine
      4. Piretanide   8. Tripamide

III. POTASSIUM SPARING DIURETICS
   a. **Aldosterone Antagonist (Aldosterone Receptor Blockers)**
      1. Spironolactone
      2. Eplerenone
      3. Canrenone
      4. Potassium canreonate
   b. **Non-Aldosterone Antagonist**
      1. Amiloride
      2. Triamterene

B. <u>OSMOTIC DIURETICS</u>
   1. Mannitol   3. Glycerine
   2. Urea   4. Isosorbide

C. <u>DRUGS INCREASING GFR/SECONDARY DIURETICS</u>
   Xanthines
      1. Aminophylline   3. Caffeine
      2. Theophylline

III. DIURETICS
(According to Efficacy)

A. **High Efficacy**
   1. Loop Diuretics
   2. Organic Mercurials

B. **Moderate Efficacy**
   1. Thiazides and Related Drugs
   2. Carbonic Anhydrase Inhibitors

C. **Low Efficacy**: Potassium Sparing Diuretics

IV. DIURETICS
(Site of Action)

(A) **Drugs Acting on Proximal Tubule**
   1. Osmotic Diuretics   4. Carbonic Anhydrase Inhibitors
   2. Acidifying Salts   5. Xanthine Diuretics
   3. Organic Mercurials   6. Metolazone

(B) Drugs Acting on Descending Limb of Loop of Henle
  Osmotic Diuretics
(C) Drugs Acting on Medullary Portion of Thick Ascending Limb of Loop of Henle
  1. Loop Diuretics   2. Organic Mercurials
(D) Drugs Acting on Cortical Portion of Thick Ascending Limb of Loop of Henle: Loop Diuretics
(E) Drugs Acting on Early Segment of Distal Tubules (Cortical Diluting Segment)
  1. Thiazides   2. Metolazone
(F) Drugs Acting on Distal Tubules
  1. Carbonic Anhydrase Inhibtors
  2. Organic mercurials (at terminal portion of distal tubules)
(G) Drugs Acting on Late Distal Tubules
  Potassium Sparing Diuretics
(H) Drugs Acting on Collecting Tubule
  1) K^+ - **Sparing Diuretics**
     a) Aldosterone Antagonists
     b) Non-Aldosterone Antagonists
  2) **ADH Antagonists**

IMPORTANTANT TRADE NAMES OF DIURETICS

DIAMOX	(Acetazolamide)
LASIX	(Furosemide)
ALDACTONE	(Spironoactone)
MODURETIC	(Amiloride & Hydrochlorthiazide)
DYAZIDE	(Triamterene)
SPIROMIDE	(Spironolactone & Frusemide)
LASORIDE	(Furosemide & Amiloride)

Potassium Sparing Diuretics and Combination Preparations

Trade name	Potassium sparing agent	Hydrochlorothiazide	Dose/day
Aldactazide	Spironolactone 25mg	25mg	1-4 times
Aldactone	Spironolactone 25mg	---	1-4 times
Dyazide	Triamterene 50mg	25mg	1-4 times
Dyrenium	Triamterene 50mg	---	1-3 times
Inspra	Eplerenone 25,50mg	---	Od or bid
Maxzide	Triamterene 75mg	50mg	Od
Maxzide25mg	Triamterene 27.5mg	25mg	Od
Midamor	Amiloride 5mg	---	Od
Moduretic	Amiloride 5mg	50mg	Od or bid

DRUGS WITH IMPORTANT ACTIONS ON SMOOTH MUSCLES
Antihistamines, Serotonin, & Ergot Alkaloids

H1-RECEPTOR ANTAGONISTS

I. H-1 Receptor Blockers (Antihistamines)

1. **Alkylamines**
   1. Chlorpheniramine maleate
   2. Pheniramine maleate
   3. Brompheniramine maleate
   4. Triprolidine HCl
   5. Dimethindine maleate
   6. Azelastine
   7. Azatadine

2. **Ethylenediamines**
   1. Antazoline HCl
   2. Mepyramine Maleate
   3. Tripellenamine Citrate
   4. Methapyrilene HCl

3. **Ethanolamines**
   1. Clemastine Fumarate
   2. Diphenhydramine HCl
   3. Dimenhydrinate

4. **Piperazines**
   1. Cyclizine HCl
   2. Chlorcyclizine
   3. Meclizine HCl
   4. Buclizine
   5. Hydroxyzine HCl

5. Phenothiazines
 1. Promethazine HCl
 2. Promethazine Theoclate
 3. Trimeprazine Tartrate
 4. Dimethothiazine Mesylate
 5. Methdilazine HCl

6. Piperidines
 1. Terphenadines
 2. Astemizole

7. Miscellaneous
 1. Cyproheptadine HCl
 2. Mebhydrolin Napadisylate
 3. Phenindamine Tartrate
 4. Diphenylpyraline HCl
 5. Clemizole

II. H-2 Blockers
 1. Cimetidine
 2. Famotidine
 3. Nizatidine
 4. Ranitidine

III. 5-HT (Hydroxytryptomine) Agonists
 1. Naratriptan
 2. Rizatriptan
 3. Sumatriptan
 4. Zolmitriptan
 5. Cisapride

IV. 5-HT Antagonists
 1. Granisetron
 2. Ondansetron

ERGOT ALKALOIDS

1. Dihydroergotamine
2. Ergonovine
3. Ergotamine (mixtures)
4. Ergotamine tartrate
5. Methylgonovine
6. Methysergide

KININS (Vasodiltor polypeptides)
1. Kallidin, a decapeptide
2. Bradykinin, a nonapeptide
3. Aprotinin

SUBSTANCE P (Undecapeptide)

EICOSANOIDS
(Prostaglandins, Thromboxanes, Leukotrienes)

1. Prostaglandins
   Dinoprostane (Prostaglandin E-2)
   Dinoprost tromethamine (Prostin E-2 alpha)
   Carboprost tromethamine (15 methyl PGF2)
   Alprostadil (Prostaglandin E1) (Prostin VR, Caverjet, Edex)
   Epoprostenol (Prostacyclin)
   Latanoprost
   Misoprostol (a synthetic analog of prostaglandin E1)
   Enprostil (a synthetic analog of prostaglandin E)

2. Thromboxanes
   TXA & TXB

3. Hydroperoxyeicosatetraenoic Acids and Hydroxyeicosatetraenoic   Acids (HETEs)

4. Leukotrienes
   Groups: LTA, LTB, LTC, LTD
   Leukotriene receptor inhibtors
      1. Monteleukast   2. Zafirlukast
   Lipoxygenase inhibitor: Zileuton

BRONCHIAL ASTHMA

A. BRONCHODILATORS
I. Sympathomimetics
1. α and β Adrenoceptor Agonists
   1. Adrenaline
   2. Ephedrine
2. β (β1 + β2) adrenoceptor Agonists
   1. Isoprenaline
   2. Orciprenaline
   3. β2 Adrenoceptor Agonists
   4. Salbutamol sulphate
   5. Terbutaline sulphate
   6. Fenoterol HBr
   7. Remiterol HCl

II. Methylxanthines
1. Aminophylline
2. Theophylline
3. Choline Theophylline
4. Diphylline
5. Oxtriphylline
6. Pentoxifylline (Intermittent claudication)

III. Muscarinic Antagonists (Antimuscarinic)
1. Atropine
2. Ipratropium Bromide
3. Tiotropium

B. CORTICOSTEROIDS
1. Hydrocortisone
2. Prednisolone
3. Betamethasone valerate
4. Beclomethasone dipropionate
5. Budesonide dexamethasone
6. Flusinolide
7. Fluticasone
8. Mometasone

C. MAST CELL STABILIZERS
1. Na Chromoglycate
2. Nedocromil sodium
3. Ketotifen

D. **LEUKOTRIENE PATHWAY INHIBITORS**

   Leukotriene Receptors Antagonist
     1. Montelukast Na
     2. Zafirlukast
   5-Lipoxygenase inhibitors: Zileuton

E. **NEW APPROACHES**

   Immunomodulants Antibodies
     1. Omalizumab (IgE antibodies)
     2. Cycloserine
   Potassium Channel Activators
     Cromakalin
   Calcium Channel Blockers
     1. Verapamil
     2. Nifedipine
     3. Nitric oxide

F. **OXYGEN THERAPY**

DRUGS USED IN ASTHMA

I. **Sympathomimetics used in Asthma**
   1. Albuterol
   2. Albuterol+Ipratropium
   3. Bitolterol
   4. Ephedrine
   5. Epinephrine
   6. Formoterol
   7. Isoetharine
   8. Isoproterenol
   9. Levalbuterol
   10. Metaproterenol
   11. Pirbuterol
   12. Salmeterol
   13. Salmeterol+Fluticasone
   14. Terbutaline

II. **Aerosol Corticosteroids**
   1. Beclomethasone
   2. Budesonide
   3. Flunisolide
   4. Fluticasone
   5. Fluticasone+Salmeterol
   6. Triamcinolone

III. Leukotriene Inhibitors
    1. Monteleukast   2. Zafirleukast
    3. Zyleuton

IV. Cromolyn Sodium & Nedocromol Sodium
    1. Cromolyn Sodium
    2. Nedocromil Sodium

V. Methylxanthines (Theophylline & Derivatives)
    1. Aminophylline (Theophylline ethylenediamine)
    2. Theophylline

VI. Other Methylxanthines
    1. Dyphilline
    2. Oxtriphylline
    3. Pentoxifylline

VII. Antimuscarinic Drugs Used In Asthma
    Ipratropium (Atrovent: Aerosol, Nasal spray)

VIII. Antibody
    Omalizumab (Xolair, powder for subcutaneous injection)

BRONCHODILATORS

I. SYMPATHOMIMETICS

    a. Selective β2 Stimulants
        1. Salbutamol sulphate
        2. Terbutaline sulphate
        3. Fenoterol HBr
        4. Isoetharine HCl
        5. Pirbuterol
        6. Reporterol HCl
        7. Rimiterol HCl
        8. Hexoprenaline

b. Drugs Stimulating β(both β1+β2) Receptors

1. Isoprenaline Sulphate
2. Orciprenaline Sulphate

c. Drugs Stimulating both α and β Receptors

1. Adrenaline   2. Ephedrine HCl

II. XANTHINE DERIVATIVES

1. Aminophylline
2. Theophylline
3. Pentifylline
4. Proxyphylline
5. Etaminphylline Camsylate
6. Choline theophyllinate
7. Acepifylline
8. Diprophylline
9. Etophylline

III. PARASYMPATHOLYTICS

1. Atropine Sulpahte
2. Atropine methylnitrate
3. Hyoscine HBr
4. Stramonium
5. Ipratropium

IV. ANTIHISTAMINES

1. Diphenhydramine
2. Promethazine HCl
3. Chlorpheniramine maleate

V. MISCELLANEOUS

1. Papavarine HCl
2. Nitrites

DRUGS THAT ACT IN THE CENTRAL NERVOUS SYSTEM

SEDATIVE-HYPNOTICS

A. Barbiturates (According to duration of action)
   1. Long-acting Barbiturates (DOA: 8-12 hours)
      1. Phenobarbitone
      2. Barbitone
      3. Methylphenobarbitone
   2. Intermediate-acting (DOA: 4-8hours)
      1. Amylobarbitone
      2. Butobarbitone
      3. Cyclobarbitone
      4. Pentobarbitone
   3. Short-acting Barbiturates (DOA: 2-4 hrs)
      Quinal barbitone
   4. Ultra-short Acting (DOA: 15-30 min)
      1. Thiopentone Sodium
      2. Methohexitone
      3. Thiamylal Hexobarbitone

B. Benzodiazepines (according to duration of action)
   1. Long Acting (DOA: 10-24 hours)
      1. Diazepam
      2. Chlorazepate
      3. Chlordiazepoxide
      3. Flurazepam
      4. Prazepam
   2. Intermediate Acting (DOA: 5-10 hours)
      1. Alprazolam
      2. Lorazepam
      3. Oxazepam
      4. Temazepam
      5. Estazolam

3. **Short-Acting (DOA: 1-3hrs)**
   Triazolam

C. **Newer Agents**
   1. Imidazopyridine derivative
      Zolpidem
      Zaleplon
   2. 5 HT_{1A} Partial agonist
      Buspirone

D. **Older agents**
   1. Paraldehyde   4. Ethyl alcohol
   2. Methaqualone   5. Glutethimide
   3. Chloral Hydrate

SEDATION-DOSAGE

Drug	Dosage
Alprazolam	0.25-0.5 mg 2-3 times daily
Buspirone	5-10 mg 2-3 times daily
Chlordiazepoxide	10-20 mg 2-3 times daily
Chlorazepate	5-7.5 mg twice daily
Diazepam	5 mg twice daily
Halazepam	20-40 mg 3-4 times daily
Lorazepam	1-2 mg once or twice daily
Oxazepam	15-30 mg 3-4 times daily
Phenobarbital	15-30 mg 2-3 times daily
Prazepam	10-20 mg 2-3 times daily

HYPNOSIS-DOSAGE

Drug	Dosage(at Bedtime)
Chloral hydrate	500-100 mg
Estazolam	0.5-2 mg
Flurazepam	15-30 mg
Lorazepam	2-4 mg
Quazepam	7.5-15 mg
Secobarbital	100-200 mg
Temazepam	7.5-30 mg
Triazolam	0.125-0.5 mg
Zaleplon	5-20 mg
Zolpidem	5-10 mg

Acute Alcohol Withdrawal Syndrome
   1. Clorazepate   4. Diazepam
   2. Lorazepam   5. Oxazepam
   3. Thiamine

Drugs for Prevention of Alcohol Abuse
   1. Disulfiram
   2. Naltrexone

Drugs for the Treatment of Acute Methanol or Ethylene Glycol Poisoning
   1. Ethanol
   2. Fomepizole

ANTI-EPILEPTIC DRUGS
(Antiseizure Drugs)

1. **HYDANTOINS**
   1. Phenytoin
   2. Mephenytoin
   3. Ethotoin Phenacemide
2. **IMINOSTILBENES**
   1. Carbamazepine
   2. Oxcarbazepine
3. **BARBITURATES & CONGENERS**
   1. Phenobarbitone
   2. Pentobarbital sodium
   3. Phenobarbital
   4. Primidone
4. **BENZODIAZEPINES**
   1. Diazepam
   2. Clonazepam
   3. Nitrazepam
   4. Chlorazepate dipotassium
5. **PHENYLTRIAZINE**
      Lamotrigine
6. **VALPROCIC ACID** (Depakene) & Valproate sodium

7. **SUBSTITUTED MONOSACCHARIDE**
   Topiramate
8. **SULFONAMIDE DERIVATIVE**
   1. Zonisamide
   2. Piracetam
   3. Levetiracetam
   4. Acetazolamide
   5. Sulthiame
9. **NEWER DRUGS**
   1. Lamotrigine
   2. Gabapentin
   3. Oxcarbazepine
   4. Topiramate
   5. Vigabatrin
   6. Levetiracetam

DRUGS USED IN INFANTILE SPASMS
1. Corticotropin: IM
2. Prednisone: IM or oral
3. Benzodiazepines
   Clonazepam
   Nitrazepam
4. Vigabatrin

GENERAL ANESTHETICS

I. Inhalational General Anaesthetics
    A. Volatile liquids
       Older G.A
        1. Ether (Diethyl ether)
        2. Chloroform
    B. Halogenated G.A
        1. Halothane
        2. Methoxyflurane
        3. Enflurane
        4. Isoflurane

    5. Desflurane
    6. Sevoflurane
C. Gases
    1. Nitrous oxide
    2. Cyclopropane
    3. Ethylene

II. Intravenous General Anaesthetics
  A. Barbiturates
    1. Thiopentone sodium
    2. Hexobarbitone
    3. Methohexital
  B. Non-Barbiturates
    1. **Phencyclidine Derivative**
       Ketamine

    2. **Benzodiazepines**
       1. Diazepam
       2. Lorazepam
       3. Midazolam

    3. **Neuroleptic Analgesia/Anaesthesia**
       Droperidol & Fentanyl

    4. **Opioid Analgesic Anaesthesia**
       1. Morphine   4. Sufentanil
       2. Fentanyl   5. Alfentanil
       3. Remifentanil
    5. **Miscellaneous Drugs**
       1. Propofol
       2. Etomidate
       3. Propanidid

III. Rectal General Anaesthetics
    1. Thiopentone sodium
    2. Paraldehyde
    3. Tribromoethanol

LOCAL ANAESTHETICS
(Chemical Classification)

A. **Esters of Benzoic Acid**
 1. Cocaine
 2. Tetracaine
 3. Benzocaine
 4. Amethocaine

A. **Esters of Paramino Benzoic Acid (PABA)**
 1. Procaine
 2. Chlorprocaine

B. **Esters of Metaamino Benzoic Acid:** Cyclomethycaine

D. **Amides**
 1. Lidocaine
 2. Mepivacaine
 3. Bupivacaine
 4. Etidocaine
 5. Prilocaine
 6. Ropivacaine
 7. Lignocaine

E. **Ethers**
 Pramoxine

F. **Ketones**
 Dyclonine

G. **Phenetidin Derivatives**
 Phenacaine

H. **Alcohol Group**   Benzyl Alcohol

LOCAL ANAESTHETICS
(Duration of Action)

A. **Short Duration of Action**
 Procaine

B. **Medium Duration of Action**
 1. Cocaine
 2. Lidocaine
 3. Mepivacaine
 4. Prilocaine

C. Long Duration of Action
  1. Tetracaine
  2. Bupivacaine
  3. Etidocaine
  4. Ropivacaine

LOCAL ANAESTHETICS
(Therapeutic Classification)

A. Only for Surface Anaesthesia
  1. Cocaine
  2. Benzocaine
  3. Cyclomethycaine
  4. Benzyl alcohol

C. Only for Injection
  1. Procaine
  2. Amethocaine
  3. Lignocaine
  4. Cinchocaine

C. For both surface & injection purpose
  1. Lidocaine
  2. Tetracaine

SKELETAL MUSCLE RELAXANTS

Non-depolarizing agents
  1. Tubocurarine
  2. Dimethyltubocurarine
  3. Gallamine
  4. Pancuronium
  5. Alcuronium
  6. Vecuronium
  7. Atracurium
  8. Fazadinium

A. Centrally Acting Muscle Relaxants
  I. Benzodiazepines
  1. Diazepam
  4. Chlordiazepoxide
  2. Ketazolam
  5. Medazepam
  3. Chlorazepate

  II. GABA Analogue
  Beclofen

  III. Propanediol Derivatives
  1. Mephenesin
  3. Styramate
  2. Carisoprodol
  4. Meprobamate

IV. **Benzoxazole Derivatives**
      1. Chlorzoxazone
      2. Benzimidazole
      3. Zoxazolamine
   V. **Miscellaneous Compounds**
      1. Chlormezanone
      2. Orphenadrine HCl
      3. Cyclobenzaprine
      4. Orphenadrine citrate
      5. Chlorphenesin
      6. Methacarbamol
B. **Peripherally Acting Muscle Relaxants**
   I. **Neuromuscular Blocking Drugs**
      1. Atracurium
      2. Doxacurium
      3. Mevacurium
      4. Pipecuronium
      5. Rocuronium
      6. Tubocurarine
      7. Cisatracurium
      8. Metocurine
      9. Pancuronium
      10. Rapacuronium
      11. Succinylcholine
      12. Vecuronium
   II. **Spasmolytics**
      1. Beclofen
      2. Carisoprodol
      3. Chlorzoxazone
      4. Dantrolene
      5. Gabapentin
      6. Methocarbamol
      7. Riluzole
      8. Botulinum toxin type A
      9. Chlorphenesin
      10. Cyclobenzprine
      11. Diazepam
      12. Metaxolone
      13. Orphenadrine
      14. Tizanidine

PARKINSONISM & OTHER MOVEMENT DISORDERS

A. **DOPAMINERGIC DRUGS**
   I. **Levodopa**
      1. Levodopa
      2. Carbidopa
      3. Carbidopa+Levodopa (Sinemet)
   II. **Dopamine Agonist**
      i. **Ergot Derivatives**
         1. Bromocriptine
         2. Pergolide

    ii. Non Ergot Derivatives
      1. Pramipexole
      2. Ropinorole
      3. Amantadine

B. MAO-B Inhibitors
   1. Selegiline   2. Rasagiline

C. COMT – Inhibitors
   1. Tolcapone   2. Entacapone

D. ANTIMUSCARINIC
   1. Benztropine mesylate 2. Orphenadrine
   3. Procyclidine   4. Trihexephenidyl

E. MISCELLANEOUS
   1. Neuroprotective agents
   2. Coenzyme Q
   3. Vit E
   4. Biperiden
   5. Penicillamine
   6. Trientine

ANTI PARKINSONISM DRUGS

I. Dopaminergic Drugs

Levodopa

Peripheral decarboxylase Inhibitors
   1. Carbidopa
   2. Benserazide

Ergolines
   1. Bromocriptene
   2. Lergotrile

Aporphines
   1. Apomorphine
   2. N-propylnoraporphine

Monoamine Oxidase β Inhibitors
   Deprenyl

Dopamine Releasing Drugs
   Amantadine HCl

Dopamine β - Hydroxylase Inhibitors
   Fusaric acid

II. Anticholinrgic Drugs
Natural Belladona Alkaloids
   1. Atropine
   2. Hyoscine
Synthetic Anticholinergics
   1. Benzhexol HCl (Trihexphenidyl)
   2. Benztropine Mesylate
   3. Biperiden HCl
   4. Procyclidine HCl
Antihistamines
   1. Diphenhydramine HCl
   2. Orphenadrine
   3. Orphenadrine Citrate
Phenothiazines with Anticholinergic Activity
   Ethpropazine HCl

ANTI-ALZEHEIMER DRUGS

I. Uncompetitive Inhibitors of Acetylcholinesterase
   1. Donepezil
   2. Rivastigmine
   3. Tacrine

II. Competitive Inhibitor of Acetylcholinesterase:
   Galantamine

III. Uncompetitive Inhibitor of NMDA Receptors:
   Memantine

PSYCHOTROPIC DRUGS

1. Antipsychotics (Major Tranquillizers)
2. Anti-Anxiety drugs (Minor Tranquillizers)
3. Anti-Depressants
4. Psychomimetic or Psychodelic Drugs

ANTIPSYCHOTIC DRUGS
Antipsychotics/MajorTranqullizers/Neuroleptics
or Anti-Schizophrenic Drugs

A. Classical/Typical Antipsychotics

  I. Phenothiazine Derivatives
    a. Aliphatic compounds
      1. Chlorpromazine
      2. Promazine
    b. Piperazine Compounds
      1. Procholorperazine
      2. Trifluperazine
      3. Perphenazine
      4. Fluphenazine
    c. Piperidine Compounds
      1. Thioridazine
      2. Mesoridazine
  II. Butyrophenone Derivatives
      1. Haloperidol
      2. Droperidol
  III. Thioxanthenes
      1. Thiothixene
      2. Flupenthixol
  IV. Rauwolfia Alkaloids
      Reserpine

B. Newer/Atypical Antipsychotics
    Miscellaneous Structures
      1. Clopazine
      2. Olanzapine
      3. Quetiapine
      4. Pimazole
      5. Sulpiride
      6. Risperidone

C. Drugs used for Manic-Depressive Disorders
    Lithium carbonate

ANTI-ANXIETY DRUGS
(Minor Tranquillizers, Anxiolytics)

I. Benzodiazepines (According to Duration of Action)

1. **Long acting (DOA: 10-24 hours)**
   1. Diazepam
   2. Chlorazepate
   3. Flurazepam
   4. Prazepam

2. **Intermediate acting (DOA: 5-10 hours)**
   1. Alprazolam
   2. Lorazepam
   3. Oxazepam
   4. Temazepam
   5. Estazolam

3. **Short-Acting (DOA: 1-3 hours)**
   Triazolam

II. OTHER SUBSTANCES
   1. Meprobamate
   2. Benzoctamine
   3. Hydroxyzine (Anti-histamine, Antiemetic, Sedative)
   4. Chlormezanone (Skeletal muscle relaxant)

BENZODIAZEPINES
(Therapeutic Classification)

I. ANXIOLYTIC (Short term use)
  a. Sustained Action
   1. Diazepan
   2. Bromazepam
   3. Clobazepam
   4. Medazepam
   5. Alprazolam
   6. Chlordiazepoxide
   7. Chlorazepate

  b. Short Duration of Action
   1. Lorazepam
   2. Oxazepam

II. Used as Hypnotics
   a. Prolonged action (may cause hangover)
      1. Nitrazepam   3. Flunitrazepam
      2. Flurazepam   4. Diazepam
   b. Short Duartion of Action (usually no hangover)
      1. Lorazepam
      2. Lometazepam
      3. Temazepam

III. Used as Antiepileptics
     1. Diazepam   3. Clonazepam
     2. Clobazepam   4. Clorazepate

IV. Used as Muscle Relaxants
     1. Diazepam   2. Clonazepam

V. Used for Oral Pre-anaesthetic Medication
     1. Diazepam
     2. Lorazepam
     3. Temazepam

VI. Drugs Producing Amnesia
     1. Diazepam
     2. Lorazepam
     3. Midazolam

VII. Used for Induction of General Anaesthesia
       Midazolam

VIII. Drugs with Greater Risk of Withdrawal Symptoms
     1. Lorazepam
     2. Oxazepam

ANTI-DEPRESSANTS

1. Tricyclic Antidepressants
2. MAO Inhibitors
3. Second Generation Antidepressants
4. Miscellaneous

1. Tricyclic Antidepressants
A. Dibenzodiazepines
1. Imipramine HCl
2. Clomipramine
3. Desipramine
4. Trimipramine
5. Lofepramine

B. Dibenzocycloheptadines
1. Amitriptyline HCl
2. Amitriptyline Embonate
3. Nortriptyline
4. Protriptyline HCl
5. Butriptyline

C. Dibenzoxazepines: Dexopin HCl
D. Dibenzothiazepines: Dothiepin HCl

2. Monoamine Oxidase (MAO) Inhibitors

A. Hydrazine Derivatives
1. Phenelzine
2. Isocarboxazid
3. Iproniazid
4. Nialamide

B. Non-Hydrazine Derivatives
1. Tranylcypromine sulphate
2. Pargyline

3. Selective Serotonin Reuptake Inhibitors (SSRI)
1. Fluoxetine
2. Paroxatine
3. Sertraline
4. Citalopram
5. Fluvoxamine

4. **Heterocyclic/Second &Third Generation Antidepressants**

    1. **Tricyclic Drugs**: Amoxapine
    2. **Tetracyclic Drugs:**
        1. Maprotiline   2. Mianserin
    3. **Bicyclic Drugs**:   Viloxazine
    4. **Monocyclic Drugs**: Tofenacin
    5. **Others**: Trazadone, Bupropion

5. **Miscellaneous**

      1. Flupenthixol
      2. Tryptaphane
      3. Alprazolam
      4. Nomifensina

PSYCHOMIMETIC
(Hallucinogens, Psychodelic Drugs)

1.   Lysergic Acid Diethylamide (LSD)
2.   Tetrahydrocannabinol

MOOD STABILIZERS

    1. Carbamazapine   3. Lithium carbonate
    2. Divalproex   4. Valproic acid

ANALGESIC

1. Narcotic Analgesics (Opiods)
1. Non - Narcotic Analgesics (NSAIDs)

NARCOTIC ANALGESICS
(According to Source)

A. Naturally Occurring Opium Alkaloids
   1. Morphine   2. Codeine

B. Semisynthetic Derivatives of Opium Alkaloids
   1. Diamorphine (Heroin)   4. Etrophine
   2. Hydromorphone   5. Oxymorphone
   3. Hydrocodone   6. Oxycodone

C. Synthetic Morphine Substitutes
     1. Pethidine & its congeners
        Fentanyl
     2. Methadone & its congeners
        d-Propoxyphene
     3. Morphinan Compounds
        Levorphanol
     4. Benzomorphan compounds
        i. Pentazocine
        ii. Phenazocine
        iii.Cyclazocine

ANALGESIC COMBINATIONS

Codeine/acetaminophen *(Tylenol)*
Codeine/aspirin *(Empirin Compound)*
Hydrocodone/acetaminophen *(Norcet, Vicodin, Lortab)*
Hydrocodone/ibuprofen *(Vicoprofen)*
Oxycodone/acetaminophen *(Percocet, Tylox)*
Oxycodone/aspirin *(Percodon)*

NARCOTIC ANALGESICS
(Agonist-antagonist Classification of Opioids)

A. Pure Agonists

1. Morphine
2. Heroin
3. Codeine
4. Fentanyl
5. Pethidine
6. Etorphine

B. Mixed Agonist – Antagonists
1. Nalorphine
2. Cyclazocine
3. Pentazocine
4. Meptazinol

C. Pure Antagonists
1. Naloxone   (t ½: 1 hour) All receptors (μ,κ,δ,σ)
2. Naltrexone (t ½: 10 hours)
3. Nalmefene

Common Opioid Analgesics

1. Morphine
2. Hydromorphone
3. Oxymorphone
4. Methadone
5. Meperidine
6. Fentanyl
7. Sufentanil
8. Alfentanil
9. Codeine
10. Hydrocodone
11. Oxycodone
12. Propoxyphene
13. Pentazocine
14. Nalbuphine
15. Buprenorphine
16. Levorphanol

CENTRAL NERVOUS SYSTEM DEPRESSANTS

1. ALIPHATIC ALCOHOLS
  1. Ethyl alcohol
  2. Methyl alcohol

2. HYPNOTICS
  1. Barbiturates
  2. Non-barbiturates

3. ANTIEPILEPTICS
   1. Sodium valproate
   2. Phenytoin
   3. Phenothiazine
   4. Carbamazapine
4. ANALGESICS-ANTIPYRETICS (Non-Narcotic)
   1. Aspirin
   2. Sodium salicylate
   3. Paracetamol
5. NARCOTICS (Narcotic Analgesics)
   Opioid analgesics: Opium (alkaloid morphine; synthetic drug: pethidine)
6. TRANQUILLIZERS (Anti-Anxiety Drugs)
   i. **Major Tranquillizers (Antipsychotics)**
      1. Chlorpromazine
      2. Reserpine
   ii. **Minor Tranquillizers**
      1. Diazepam
      2. Chlordiazepoxide
7. LOCAL ANAESTHETICS
   1. Cocaine
   2. Procaine
8. GENERAL ANAESTHETICS
   i. Volatile Liquids
   ii. Gases
   iii. Intravenous Anaesthetics

DRUGS OF ABUSE

1. **Opioids**
   Intraveous use, intranasal use, oral use and smoking of heroin
2. **Sedative-Hypnotics**
   1. Barbiturates
   2. Benzodiazepines
   3. Alcohol
   4. Gamma-hydroxybutyric acid (GHB)

3. Stimulants
1. Caffeine
2. Nicotine
3. Cocaine
4. Amphetamine
5. Analogs of amphetamine
   Methylphenidate
   Methylenedioxymethamphetamine (MDMA)
   Cathinone

4. Hallucinogens
1. LSD-like group of drugs
   Lysergic acid diethylamide (LSD)
   Mescaline (phenethylamine derivative)
   Psilocybin (indolethylamine derivative)
2. Phencyclidine (PCP,angel dust):a veterinary anaesthetic
3. Ketamine (analog of Phencyclidine)

5. Deliriant Hallucinogens
1. Scopolamine
2. Synthetic centrally acting cholinoceptor blocking agents
3. Anticholinergic antiparkinsonism drugs
4. Tricyclic antidepressants
5. Antispasmodics

6. Marijuana (Cannabis)

7. Inhalants
Anaesthetic gases
Industrial solvents: Hydrocarbons like toluene
Aerosol propelleants: Fluorocarbons
Organic nitrites: Amyl or isobutyl nitrite

8. Steroids: Anabolic steroids used in competitive sports

DISEASES OF BLOOD, INFLAMMATION, AND GOUT

ANEMIAS, HEMATOPOIETIC GROWTH FACTORS
1. Iron
2. Vitamin B 12
3. Folic acid
4. Hematopoietic Growth Factors
    Erythropoietin (epoetin alfa)
    Myeloid growth factors
    Granulocyte colony-stimulating factors (G-CSF)
    Granulocyte macrophage colony-stimulating factor (GM-CSF)
    Megakaryocyte growth facctors
    Interleukin-11

COMMONLY USED ORAL IRON PREPARATIONS
(Dosage: 200-400 mg/day for 3-6 months)

Preparation	Tablet size	Elemental iron per tablet	Usual adult dosage (tablets per day)
Ferrous sulfate, hydrated	325 mg	65 mg	3-4
Ferrous sulfate, dessicated	200 mg	65 mg	3-4
Ferrous gluconate	325 mg	36 mg	3-4
Ferrous fumarate	200 mg	66 mg	3-4
Ferrous fumarate	325 mg	106 mg	2-3

HEMOSTATICS
(Coagulants)

I. SYSTEMIC HEMOSTATICS
  a. Antifibrinolytic (Inhibitors of Plasmin Activators)
    Aminocaproic Acid
    Tranxamic Acid
  b. Proteolytic enzyme Inhibitors (Plasmin Inhibitors)
    Aprotinin
  c. By Correcting Abnormal Platelet Adhesion
    Ethamsylate
  d. Agents which Augment Coagulation Factor Synthesis
    Vitamin K Preparations
      Phytomenadione (Vit.K1)
      Menadione (Vit.K3)
      Menadione Sodium Bisulphate
      Menadione Sodium Phosphate
  e. Agents that Overcome Specific Coagulation Defects
    Antihaemophilic Factor (Factor, AHF)
    Cryoprecipitated Antihaemophilic Factor
    Factor IX Complex (Plasma Thromboplastin Component)

II. LOCAL HAEMOSTATICS
  a. Absorbable Agents Assisting Fibrin Formation
    Oxidised Cellulose
    Absorbable Gelatin Sponge (Gelfoam)
    Oxidised Regenerated Cellulose (Surgical)
    Microfibrillar collagen Haemostat
    Calcium Alginate
  b. Vasoconstrictors
    1. Adrenaline   2. Noradrenaline
  c. Astringents
    1. Alum   2. Iron salts
  d. Blood Preparations
    1. Thrombin   2. Fibrinogen
    3. Fibrin

ANTICOAGULANTS

I. Used in both Vivo and Vitro.
    Heparin sodium

II. Used in Vivo only
    Coumarin Derivatives
      Warfarin
        Dicumarol
      Nicoumalone
        Phenprocoumon
    Indandione Derivatives
      Phenidione
      Diphendione
      Anisindione

III. Used in Vitro only
    Oxalates and Citrates of Na^+ and K^+
      i. K-oxalate
      ii. Na-oxalate
      iii. EDTA (Ethylene Diamine Tetra Acetic Acid)
      iv. Hirudine

ANTICOAGULANTS

A. <u>Parenteral Anticoagulants</u>
  I. Indirect Thrombin Inhibitors
    a. Heparin (Sodium or Calcium Salt)
      1. Unfractionated Heparin (UFH)
      2. Low-molecular weight Heparin (LMWH)
      3. Enonaparin
      4. Dalteparin
      5. Tinzaparin
    b. Fondaparinux (Arixtra)
  II. Direct Thrombin Inhibitors (DTI)
    1. Hirudine
    2. Lepirudin

3. Bivalirudin
4. Argatroban
5. Melagatrin

B. Oral Anticoagulants
1. **Coumarin Derivatives**
   1. Warfarin Sodium (only used)
   2. Warfarin Potassium
   3. Nicoumalone
   4. Dicumoral
   5. Phenprocoumon
2. **Indendione Derivatives (not used)**
   1. Phenindione
   2. Diphenadione
   3. Anisidione
3. **Ximlagatran**
4. **Miscellaneous**
   1. By Removal of ionic Calcium Sodium Acid Citrate (an ingredient of "whole human blood" for transfusion)
   2. Potassium Oxalate
   3. Sodium Oxalate

FIBRINOLYTICS
(Thrombolytic Drugs)

1. Streptokinase
2. Urokinase
3. Stanozolol

ANTIPLATELET DRUGS
(Antithrombotic Drugs)

1. Aspirin
2. Sulphinpyrazone
3. Dipyridamole

ANTILIPIDEMIC DRUGS

I. Drugs which Alter Lipoprotein Production
   a. Clofibrate Group (Fibric acid derivatives)
      1. Clofibrate
      2. Bezafibrate
      3. Gemifibrozil
      4. Fenofibrate
   b. Nicotinic Acid Group
      1. Nicotinic Acid
      2. Nicofuranose
      3. Acipimox

II. Drugs which Decrease Absorption of Cholesterol in the gut by binding Bile Salts (Anion –Exchange Resins)
      1. Cholestyramine
      2. Colestipol

III. Drugs which Increase Catabolism of Low Density Lipoproteins
      Probucol

IV. HMG CoA Reductase Inhibitors (Statins)
      1. Simvastatin
      2. Pravastatin
      3. Lovastatin
      4. Atorvastatin
      5. Cerivastatin
      6. Fluvastatin

V. Inhibitors of Intestinal Sterol Absorption
      Ezetimibe

VI. Miscellaneous Drugs
      1. Dextrothyroxine
      2. Neomycin
      3. Oestrogens
      4. Sitosterols
      5. Sunflower oils
      6. Fish oils: Omega-3 Marine Triglycerides

7. Niacin
8. Vitamin B-3

VII. Treatment with Drug Combinations
1. Fibric Acid Derivatives & Bile Acid-Binding Resins
2. HMG-CoA Reductase & Bile Acid-Binding Resins
3. Niacin & Bile Acid-Binding Resins
4. Niacin & Reductase Inhibitors
5. Reductase Inhibitors & Ezetimibe
6. Ternary Combination of Resins, Niacin & Reductase Inhibitors

NON-STEROIDAL ANTI-INFLAMMATORY DRUGS (NSAIDs)

1. **Drug with Analgesic & Weak Anti-inflammatory Effect**
   Aniline Derivative … Acetaminophen (Paracetamol)
2. **Drugs with Analgesic & Mild to Moderate Anti-inflammatory Effect**
   a. **Propionic Acid Derivatives**
      1. Fenbufen
      2. Flurbiprofen
      3. Indoprofen
      4. Naproxen
      5. Suprofen-Tiaprofenic Acid
      6. Fenoprofen
      7. Ibuprofen
      8. Ketoprofen

   b. **Fenamic Acid Derivatives**
      1. Mefenamic Acid
      2. Flufenamic Acid
      3. Meclofenamic Sodium
3. **Drugs with Analgesic & marked Anti-inflammatory Effect**
   a. **Salicylic Acid Derivatives**
      1. Aspirin (Acetylsalicylic Acid)
      2. Salicylic Acid
      3. Sodium Salicylate
      4. Methyl Salicylate
      5. Sodium Thiosalicylate
      6. Choline Magnesium Trisalicylate
      7. Salsalate, Salicylic Acid

8. Diflunisal
9. Benorylate
10. Sulfasalazine
11. Olsalazine

b. Pyrazolone Derivatives
Azapropazone, Phenylbutazone
Oxyphenbutazone

c. Acetic Acid Derivatives
1. Diclofenac
2. Etodolac
3. Indomethacin
4. Sulindac
5. Tolmetin
6. Fenclofenac

d. Oxicam Derivatives
Piroxicam

e. COX-II Inhibitors
Celecoxib, Etodolac, Etoricoxib, Rofecoxib, Nimuselide

f. Miscellaneous:
Nabumetone
Gabatrin

DISAESE-MODIFYING ANTIRHEUMATIC DRUGS (DMARDs)

1. **Methotrexate** (By inhibition of aminoimidazole carboxamide transformylase & thymidylate synthetase)
2. **Chlorambucil** (By preventing cell replication)
3. **Cyclophosphamide** (By preventing cell replication)
4. **Cyclosporine** (By preventing cell replication)
5. **Azathioprine** (By suppression of cell function)
6. **Mycophenolate Mofetil**(MMF)(By preventing cell replication)
7. **Chloroquine and Hydroxychloroquine** (By suppression of cell function)
8. **Gold compounds** (By suppression of cell function)
    a. Parenteral
    Gold Sodium Aurothiomalate
    Aurothioglucose
    b. Oral: Auranofin

9. **Penicillamine** (Rarely used because of its toxicity)
10. **Sulfasalazine** (By suppression of cell function & replication)
11. **TNF-α Blocking Drugs** (By suppression of cell function)
    Adilamumab
    Infliximab
    Entanercept
12. **Leflunomide** (By preventing cell replication)
13. **Glucocorticoid Drugs**
14. **Immunoabsorption Apheresis** of 1200 ml of plasma weekly for 3 months (By regulation of B cell function)

DRUGS USED IN GOUT

A. Drugs Which Reduce the Production of Uric Acid
   Allopurinol

B. Drugs Which Increase Urinary Excretion of Uric Acid (Uricosuric Agents)
   1. Probenecid
   2. Sulfinpyrazone

C. NSAIDs (Inhibit prostaglandin synthase and urate crystal phagocytosis)

   1. Indomethacin
   2. Phenylbutazone
   3. Oxyphenbutazone
   4. Aspirin
   5. Sodium Salicylate
   6. Colchicine (by inhibition of leukocyte migration and phagocytosis and formation of leukotriene B4)
   7. Oxaprozin: By increaesing uric acid excretion in urine
   8. Successful treatment of Acute gouty episodes:
      All NSAIDs except Aspirin, Salicylates and Tolmetin
   9. All other NSAIDs

ENDOCRINE DRUGS

HYPOTHALAMIC & ANTERIOR PITUIATRY HORMONES

1. Bromocriptine
2. Chorionic gonadotropin (hCG)
3. Cosyntropin
4. Follitropin alfa
5. Ganirelix
6. Goserelin acetate
7. Leuprolide
8. Nafarelin
9. Protirelin
10. Sermorelin, GHRH
11. Somatotropin
12. Vasopressin
13. Cabergoline
14. Corticotropin (ACTH)
15. Thyrotropin alpha
16. Follitropin beta, FSH
17. Gonadorelin acetate
18. Histrelin
19. Menotropins, hMG
20. Octreotide
21. Pergolide
22. Somatrem
23. Somatostatin
24. Urofollitropin

POSTERIOR PITUIATRY HORMONES

1. Desmopressin
2. Oxytocin
3. Vasopressin (ADH)

HYPOTHYROIDISM
(Thyroid Agents)

1. Levothyroxine (T4)
2. Liothyronine (T3)
3. Thyroid desiccated (Thyroid powder)
4. Liotrix (4:1of T4:T3)
5. Thyrotropin (Recombinant human TSH)

HYPERTHYROIDISM
(Antithyroid Agents)

I. Thionamides
   1. Propylthiouracil   3. Carbimazole
   2. Methylthiouracil   4. Methimazole

II. Anion Inhibitors
   1. Potassium Perchlorate   2. Thiocyanate

III. Iodides
   Lugol's Iodine (Iodine 5%+Potassium Iodide10%)
   Potassium Iodide solution (Lugol's solution; Pima)

IV. Radioactive Iodine
   ^{131}I (Iodotope)

V. Iodinated Contrast Media
   1. Ipanoic acid
   2. Diatrizoate
   3. Ipodate Sodium

VI. Adjunctive Agents
   1. Beta Blockers (Adrenoceptor-blocking agents)
      1. Nadolol   2. Propranolol
   2. Diltiazem
   3. Corticosteroids
      1. Hydrocortisone   2. Dexamethasone
   4. Cholestyramine
   5. Barbiturates

THYROID STORM (Thyrotoxic Crisis)

1. **Propranolol**: 1-2 mg slowly IV or 40-80 mg orally every 6 hours
2. **Diltiazem**: 90-120 mg orally 3-4 times/day or 5-10 mg/hour by IV infusion (asthmatic patients only)
3. **Potassium iodide** (saturated solution): 10 drops orally daily or
4. **Sodium iodate**: (iodinated contrast media): 1 g orally daily
5. **Propylthiouracil**: 250 mg orally every 6 hours or 400 mg per rectum 6 hourly
6. **Methimazole**: 60 mg/day per rectum
7. **Hydrocortisone**:50 mg IV,6 hourly

NON-TOXIC GOITRE

1. Due to Iodide Deficiency
   Iodide orally: 150-200 mcg/day
   Iodized salt and iodate used in flour and bread as preservative
   Iodized poppy seed oil, through IM route (a long term source)
2. Due to Goitrogens in Diet
   Elimination of goitrogens
   Adding sufficient thyroxine to shut off TSH stimulation
3. Hashimoto's Thyroiditis and Dyshormogenesis
   Thyroxine: 150-200 mcg/day orally

ADRENOCORTICOSTEROIDS
(According to Source)

A. NATURAL
  I. Glucocorticoids
       Cortisol (Hydrocortisone)
       Corticosterone
  II. Mineralocorticoids
       11-Desoxy Corticosterone Acetate
       Aldosterone

B. SYNTHETIC
  I. Glucocorticoids(Effects on intermediary metabolism)
       1. Cortisone
       2. Prednisone
       3. Prednisolone
       4. Methyl Predinsolone
       5. Paramethasone
       6. Dexamethasone
       7. Triamcinolone
       8. Low Activity: Betamethasone Valerate
                      Beclomethasone Dipropionate
  II. Mineralocorticoid (Salt retaining activity)
       1. Fludrocortisone (Florinef acetate)
       2. Desoxycorticosterone acetate

ADRENOCORTICOSTEROIDS
(According to Duration of Activity)

I. Short to Medium-acting Glucocorticoids
1. Hydrocortisone (Cortisol)
2. Cortisone
3. Prednisone
4. Prednisolone
5. Methylprednisone
6. Meprednisone

II. Intermediate-acting Glucocorticoids
1. Triamcinolone   2. Paramethasone
3. Fluprednisolone

III. Long-acting Glucocorticoids
1. Betamethasone   2. Dexamethasone

IV. Mineralocorticoids
1. Fludrocortisone   2. Desoxycorticosterone acetate

ADRENOCORTICAL ANTAGONISTS

I. Synthesis inhibitors & Glucocorticoid Antagonists
1. Metyrapone
2. Aminoglutethimide
3. Ketoconazole
4. Mifepristone
5. Mitotane
6. Trilostane

II. Mineralocorticoid Antagonists
1. Progesterone
2. Spironolactone
3. Eplerenone
4. Drospirenone

GLUCOCORTICOIDS
(According to duration of action)

A. SHORT TO MEDIUM ACTING (Half life: 8-24 hours)
1. Cortisol
2. Cortisone
3. Prednisone
4. Prednisolone
5. Methylprednisolone
6. Meprednisone

B. INTERMEDIATE ACTING (Half life: 24 –36 hours)
1. Triamcinolone
2. Paramethasone
3. Fluprednisone

C. LONG ACTING (Half life: 36-72 hours)
1. Betamethasone
2. Dexamethasone
3. Dexamethazone acetate

GONADAL HORMONES & INHIBITORS

I. ESTROGENS
1. Conjugated estrogens
2. Dienestrol
3. Diethylstilbestrol (DES)
4. Diethylstilbestrol diphosphate
5. Esterified estrogens
6. Estradiol cypionate in oil
7. Estradiol
8. Estradiol transdermal
9. Estradiol valerate in oil
10. Estrone aqueous suspension
11. Estropipate
12. Ethinyl estradiol

II. PROGESTINS
1. Hydroxyprogesterone caproate

2. Levonorgestrel
3. Medroxyprogesterone acetate
4. Megestrol acetate
5. Norethindrone acetate
6. Norgestrel
7. Progesterone

GONADAL HORMONES
Antagonists & Inhibitors
1. Anastrozole
2. Bicalutamide
3. Clomiphene
4. Danazol
5. Exemestane
6. Finasteride
7. Flutamide
8. Letrozole
9. Nilutamide
10. Raloxifene
11. Tamoxifen
12. Toremifene

ANDROGENS & ANABOLIC STEROIDS
1. Fluoxymesterone
2. Methyltestosterone
3. Nandrolone decanoate
4. Nandrolone phenpropionate
5. Oxandrolone
6. Oxymetholone
7. Stanozolol
8. Tetsolactone
9. Testosterone aqueous
10. Testosterone cypionate in oil
11. Testosterone enanthate in oil
12. Testosterone propionate in oil
13. Testosterone transdermal system

PANCREATIC HORMONES AND ANTI-DIABETIC DRUGS

PANCREATIC HORMONE: Glucagon

ANTI-DIABETIC DRUGS

I. INSULIN

Pharmacokinetic type	Species Type	Peak DOA-hours	Activity-hours
1. Ultra short acting Insulin Lispro	Human, modified	0.25-0.5	3-4 hours
2. Short-acting Insulin Injections USP (regular, crystalline zinc)	Human, Pork	0.5-3	5-7 hours
3. Intermediate-acting -NPH insulin (Isophane insulin suspensionUSP)	Human, Pork	8-12 hours	18-24 hours
-Lente Insulin (Insulin zinc suspension USP)	Human, Pork	8-12 hours	18-24 hours
4. Long-acting -Ultra lente insulin	Human	8-12 hours	18-28 hours
5. Ultra long acting Insulin Glargine	Human, modified	No peak	> 24 hours

INSULIN PREPARATIONS

Preparation	Species source	Concentration
1. Rapid acting insulins		
Insulin lispro, Humalog(Lily)	Human analog	U100
Insulin Aspart, Novolog (Novo Nordisk)	Human analog	U100
2. Short acting insulins		
Regular (Novo Nordisk)	Human	U100
Regular Humulin(Lily)	Human	U100-U500
Velosulin BR(Novo Nordisk)	Human	U100
3. Intermediate acting insulins		
Lente Humulin(Lily)	Human	U100
Lente(Novo NorDisk)	Huamn	U100
NPH Humulin(Lily)	Human	U100
NPH(Novo NorDisk)	Human	U100
4. Premixed insulins (%NPH,%regular)		
Novolin70/30 (Novo NorDisk)	Human	U100
Humulin70/30 and 50/50(Lily)	Human	U100
Premixed (%NP-analog, %rapid acting analog)	Human analog	U100
50/50 NPL,Lispro(Lily)	Human analog	U100
75/25 NPL,Lispro,Lily	Human analog	U100
70/30 NPA,Aspart (NovoNordisk)	Human analog	U100
5. Long-acting insulins		
Ultralente Humulin U(Lily)	Human	U100
Insulin glargine-lantus(Aventis/ Hoechst Marion Roussel)	Human	U100

II. ORAL ANTIDIABETIC DRUGS

A. INSULIN SECRETOGOGUES

I. Sulfonylureas

1st Generation

1. Tolbutamide   (DOA: 6-12 hours)
2. Chlorpropamide   (DOA: Upto 60 hours)
3. Tolazomide   (DOA: 10-14 hours)

2nd Generation

1. Glyburide/Glibenclamide   (DOA: 10-24 hrs)
2. Glipizide/Glidiazinamide (DOA: 10-24 hours)
3. Glimepiride   (DOA: 12-24 hours)

II. Meglitinides: Repaglinide   (DOA: 5-8 hours)

III. D-Phenylalanine derivative

Nateglinide   (DOA: Less then 4 hours)

B. Biguanides

1. Metformin
2. Phenformin

C. Thiazolidinediones (Tzds)-by decreasing insulin resistance

1. Pioglitazone
2. Rosiglitazone

D. α-Glucosidase inhibitor

1. Acarbose
2. Miglitol

BONE MINERAL HOMEOSTASIS

I. VITAMIN D METABOLITES & ANALOGS

1. Calciferol
2. Calcitrol (Rocaltrol-oral; Calcijex-parenteral)
3. Cholecalciferol (Vitamin D-3)
4. Dihydrotachysterol (DHT)
5. Doxercalciferol
6. Ergocalciferol (Vitamin D-2)
7. Paricalcitrol

II. CALCIUM

1. Calcium Acetate
2. Calcium Carbonate
3. Calcium Chloride
4. Calcium Citrate
5. Calcium Glubionate
6. Dibasic Calcium Phosphate Dihydrate
7. Tricalcium Phosphate
8. Calcium Lactate
9. Calcium Gluconate
10. Calcium Gluceptate

III. PHOSPHATE & PHOSPHATE BINDER

1. Phosphate (Fleet phospho soda)
2. Sevelamer

IV. OTHER DRUGS

1. Alendronate
2. Calcitonin-Salmon
3. Etidronate
4. Gallium Nitrate
5. Pamidronate
6. Plicamycin
8. Tiludronate
7. Risedronate
9. Sodium Fluoride

CHEMOTHERAPEUTIC DRUGS

1. Antibiotics

    i.   Beta-Lactam Antibiotics and other Inhibitors of Cell Wall Synthesis
    ii. Chloramphenicol
    iii. Tetracyclines
    iv. Macrolides
    v.   Clindamycin
    vi. Oxazolidones
    vii. Streptogramins
    viii. Aminoglycosides and Spectinomycin
    ix. Sulfonamides, Trimethoprim, and Quinilones
    x.   Polypeptide Antibitics
    xi. Glycopeptide Antibiotics
    xii. Miscellaneous Antibiotics

2. Anti-Mycobacterial Drugs
3. Anti-Fungal Drugs
4. Anti-Viral Agents
5. Miscellaneous Antimicrobial Agents; Disifnectants, Antiseptics, & Sterilants
6. Anti-Protozoal Drugs
7. Anthelmintic Drugs
8. Cancer Chemotherapy
9. Immunopharmacology

ANTIBIOTICS

I. BETA-LACTAM ANTIBIOTICS AND OTHER INHIBITORS OF CELL WALL SYNTHESIS

A. PENICILLINS
I. Narrow Spectrum Penicillins
a. **Short Acting Penicillins(Natural Penicillins)**
  i. Benzylpenicillin
  ii. Phenoxymethylpenicillin
  iii. Phenethicillin

b. **Long Acting Penicillins**
  i. Procaine penicillin
  ii. Benethamine penicillin
  iii. Benzathine penicillin

c. **Penicillinase Resistant Penicillins**
  i. Antistaphylococcal Penicillins
  1. Cloxacillin
  2. Flucloxacillin
  3. Methicillin (Not used due to nephrotoxicity)
  4. Dicloxacillin
  5. Oxacillin
  6. Nafcillin

  ii. Penicillins against penicillinase producing Gram-Negative Bacteria except Pseudomonas
   Timocillin

II. Broad Spectrum Penicillins
1. Ampicillin
2. Amoxicillin
3. Bacampicillin
4. Pivampicillin
5. Talampicillin
6. Mezlocillin
7. Ciclacillin

Broad spectrum Penicillins Combinations
  i. Combination of Amoxycillin with Potassium Clavulanate
  Co-Amoxiclav

    ii. Combination of Ampicillin with Flucloxacillin
        Co-Fluampicil
    iii. Combination of Ampicillin with Sulbactam
    iv. Combination of Ticarcillin with Clavulanic Acid
III. **Mecillinams** (Active against Gram-negative bacteria excluding P aeruginosa)
        i. Mecillinam
        ii. Pivmecillinam
IV. **Antipseudomonal Penicillins**
    a. *Carboxypenicillins*
        Carbenicillin
        Carfecillin
    b. *Ureidopenicillins*
        Azlocillin
        Piperacillin
        Combination of Piperacillin with Tazobactams

B. **CEPHALOSPORINS AND OTHER BETA LACTAM DRUGS**
1. **Narrow Spectrum (1st Generation) Cephalosporins**
    i. **Oral**
        1. Cephadroxil
        2. Cephalexin, Cephradine
        3. Cephapirin (Parenteral & Oral)
        4. Cephradine (Parenteral & Oral)
    ii. **Parenteral**
        1. Cefazolin
        2. Cephalothin
2. **Intermediate Spectrum (2nd Generation) Cephalosporins**
    i. **Oral**
        1. Cefaclor
        2. Cefpodoxime proxetil
        3. Cefprozil
        4. Cefuroxime axetil
    ii. **Parenteral**
        1. Cefamandole
        2. Cefmetazole

3. Cefonicid
4. Ceforanide
5. Cefotetan
6. Cefoxitin
7. Cefuroxime
3. **Broad-Spectrum (3rd & 4th-Generation) Cephalosporins**
   i. **Oral**
      Cefixine
   ii. **Parenteral**
      Cefoperazone
      Cefotaxime
      Ceftazidime
      Ceftizoxime
C. **OTHER DRUGS**
   1. Cycloserine   2. Fosfomycin
   3. Vancomycin

II. **CHLORAMPHENICOL**   Chloromycetin
III. **TETRACYCLINES**
   i. **Short acting (6-8 hours)**
      1. Tetracycline   4. Chlortetracycline
      2. Oxytetracycline   5. Lymecycline
      3. Rolitetracycline
   ii. **Intermediate acting (9-12 hours)**
      1. Demeclocycline
      2. Methacycline
   iii. **Long acting (15-12 hours)**
      1. Doxycycline   2. Minocycline
IV. **MACROLIDES**
   1. Azithromycin   3. Erythromycin
   2. Clarithromycin   4. Spiramycin
V. **CLINDAMYCIN**
VI. **STREPTOGRAMINS**
   Quinupristin+dalfopristin (Synercid)
VII. **OXAZOLIDONES:**   Linezolid
VIII. **AMINOGLYCOSIDES AND SPECTINOMYCIN**

   1. Amikacin   6. Gentamicin

2. Kanamycin
3. Netilmicin
4. Spectinomycin
5. Tobramycin
7. Neomycin sulphate
8. Paromomycin
9. Streptomycin

IX. SULFONAMIDES, TRIMETHOPRIMS, & QUINOLONES
General-Purpose Sulfonamides
1. Multiple sulfonamides, trisulfapyrimidines
2. Sulfadiazine
3. Sulfamethizole
4. Sulfamethoxazole
5. Sulfisoxazole

Sulfonamides for Special Application
1. Mafenide
2. Sulfasalazine
3. Silver sulfadiazine
4. Sulfacetamide solution

Trimethoprim
1. Trimethoprim
2. Trimethoprim+sulfamethoxazole (Co-trimxoazole)

Quinilones & Fluoroquinolones
1. Cinoxacin
2. Enoxacin
3. Levofloxacin
4. Moxifloxacin
5. Norfloxacin
6. Sparfloxacin
2. Ciprofloxacin
8. Gatifloxacin
9. Lomefloxacin
10. Nalodixic acid
11. Ofloxacin
12. Travofloxacin

X. POLYPEPETIDE ANTIBIOTICS
Polymyxins
1. Polymyxin-B Sulphate (Parenteral, Ophthalmic)
2. Colistin (Polymyxin E)
3. Bacitracin

XI. GLYCOPEPTIDE ANTIBIOTICS
1. Vancomycin
2. Teicoplanin

XI. MISCELLANEOUS ANTIBIOTICS
1. Novobiocin
3. Lincomycin
3. Fucidic acid and its salt Sodium Fucidate
4. Clindamycin
5. Spectinomycin

MISCELLANEOUS ANTIMICROBIAL DRUGS

1. Methenamine hippurate
2. Metronidazole
3. Polymyxin B (Polymixin B sulphate)
4. Methanamine mandelate
5. Nitrofurantoin

Bacteriostatic and Bactericidal Antibacterial Agents

Bactericidal agents	Bacteriostatic agents
Aminoglycosides	Chloramphenical
Bacitracin	Clindamycin
Beta-lactam antibiotics	Ethambutol
Isoniazid	Macrolides
Metronidazole	Nitrofurantoin
Polymyxins	Novobiocin
Pyrazinamide	Oxazolidinones
Quinolones	Sulfonamides
Quinupristin-dalfopritin	Tetracyclines
Rifampacin	Trimethoprim
Vancomycin	

ANTIVIRAL AGENTS
(Mechanism of Action)

I. **Inhibitors of Adsorption and Penetration of Susceptible Cells**
   1. Gamma Globulin
   2. Amantadine
   3. Rimantadine
II. **Inhibitors of Intracellular Synthesis**
   a. *Inhibitors of early protein synthesis*
      1. Guanidine
      2. Hydroxybenzyl benzimidazole
   b. *Inhibitors of nucleic acid synthesis*
      1. Ribavirin
      2. Pyrimidines and purine analogue
         i. 5 Fu   5 Bu
         ii. Idoxuridine

       iii. Cytarabine
       iv. Vidarabine (Vira-A)
   3. Other inhibitors of nucleic acid synthesis
       i. Foscarnet
       ii. Phosphonoacetic acid
       iii. Acyclovir
       iv. Ganiclovir
       v. Dideoxynucleosides
       vi. Dideoxycytidine
       vii. Interferones
           Interferon alfa-2a
           Interferon alfa-2b
           Interferon alfa-2b
           Interferon alfa-n3
           Interferon alfacon-1
           Interferon beta-1a
           Interferon beta-1b

III. Inhibitors of Late Protein Synthesis
   1. Fluorphenylalanine
   2. Puromycin
   3. Methisazone

IV. Inhibitors of Assembly or Release of Viral Particles
   1. 5-fluro 2-deoxyuridine
   2. Puromycin
   3. Rifampin

ANTIVIRAL AGENTS
(Therapeutic Classification)

I. Used against Respiratory Infections
   1. Amantadine   3. Rimantadine
   2. Ribavarin   4. Interferon

II. To Prevent or Treat Herpes Simplex Virus (HSV) and Varicella Zoster Virus (VZV)
   1. Acyclovir   6. Foscarnet

2. Famciclovir
3. Ganiclovir
4. Peciclovir
5. Valacyclovir (topical)
7. Vidarabine
8. Idoxuridine
9. Trifluridine (topical)

III. Agents to Treat Cytomegalovirus (CMV) Infections
1. Cidofovir
2. Foscarnet
3. Valgancyclovir
4. Fomivirsen
5. Ganciclovir

IV. Used against Human Immunodeficiency Virus (HIV)
Zidovudine (Azidothymidine)(AZT)

V. Used against Viral Hepatitis
Hepatitis B
1. Lamivudine
2. Adefovir
3. Interferon alfa-2b

Hepatitis C
1. Interferon alfa-2b
2. Interferon alfa-2a
3. Interferon alfacon-1
4. Pegylated interferon alfa-2a
5. Pegylated interferon alfa-2b

VI. Anti-influenzal agents
1. Amantadine
2. Rimantadine

VII. Anti-retroviral Agents
Abacavir (NRTI)
Amprenavir (Protease inhibitors)
Delavirdine (NNRTI)
Didanosine (NRTI)
Protease inhibitors
Efavirenz (NNRTI)
Enfuvirtide& Lopinavir/ritonavir
Indinavir (Protease inhibitors)
Lemivudine (NRTI)
Nelfinavir (Protease inhibitors)
Nevirapene (NNRTI)
Ritonavir (Protease inhibitors)
Saquinavir hard gel, & soft gel-
Stavudine (NRTI)
Tenofovir
Zalcitabine (NRTI)
Zidovudine (NRTI)
Zidovudine plus Lamivudine (NRTI)

DISINFECTANTS, ANTISEPTICS AND STERILANTS

1. **ALCOHOLS** (Antiseptics & Disinfectants)
    1. Ethyl alcohol (Ethanol) 10%
    2. Isopropyl alcohol (isopropanol) 70-90%
    3. Industrial methylated spirit

2. **ALDEHYDES** (Reducing agents) (Disinfectant, Sterilant)
    1. Formaldehyde solution 37% (Formalin)
    2. Glutaraldehyde

3. **ACIDS** (Inorganic and Organic)
    1. Boric acid 5%(Inorganic)
    2. Benzoic acid 0.1%
    3. Acetic acid 0.25-2%
    4. Salicylic acid
    5. Mandelic acid

4. **HALOGENS AND HALOGENS CONTAINING COMPOUNDS**
   Iodine (Bactericidal, Antiseptic)
   Lugol's solution (Iodine aqueous)
   Tincture iodine
   Povidine-iodine (Betadine)
   Iodophors: Polyvinyl pyrrolidone (Antiseptics & Disinfectants)
   Chlorine: (Disinfectants)(Chlorine containing compounds)
    1. Chloramine (Halazone)
    2. Sodium hypochlorite (Dakin's solution)

5. **OXIDIZING AGENTS** (Peroxygen Compounds)
    1. Hydrogen peroxide (bactericial, sporicidal, fungicidal, viricidal)
    2. Hydrogen Peroxide 3%
    3. Sodium Perborate
    4. Potassium permanganate (1:10,000)
    5. Zinc Peroxide
    6. Peracetic Acid

6. HEAVY METAL SALTS (Disinfectants)
Mercury Compounds
Mercuric Chloride
Ammoniated Mercury (Hg NH_2 Cl)
Phenylmercuric Nitrate/Acetate
Thimerosal(Preservative in vaccines, antitoxins & immune sera)
Merbromin (Mercurochrome)
Silver Compounds: Silver Nitrate
(Inorganic Silver Salts are strongly bactericidal, silver nitrate 1:1000 was used as prenetive for gonococcal ophthalmitis in newborn).
Silver Protein (Argyrol SS 10%)
Zinc Compounds
Zinc Oxide
Zinc Peroxide
Zinc Sulphate

7. PHENOLS AND ITS DERIVATIVES
Derivatives (Antiseptic & Disinfectants): Bactericidal, fungicidal, inactivates lipophilic viruses (for disinfection of floors, beds, counter or bench tops)

1. Cresol
2. Phenol (Carbolic acid)
3. Thymol
4. Hexa chlorophene (pH isohex, Septisol)
5. Chlorhexidine gluconate (Hibiclenz, Hibistat)
6. Chloroxylenol
7. Xylenols
8. Resorcinol
9. Hexylresorcinol

8. SYNTHETIC ORGANIC DYES
1. Acriflavine
2. Gentian violet
3. Methylene blue

9. MISCELLANEOUS
Surface – active agents (Surfactant-Detergents)
1. Anionic surface-active agents: Soft soap
2. Cationic surface-active agents
    i. Benzalkonium Chloride (Zephiran)
    ii. Cetyl Pyridinum Chloride
    iii. Cetrimide

3. Icthamol
4. Coal Tar

Quaternary Ammonium Compounds (Quarts): (Bacteriostatic, fungistatic, sporistatic, inhibit algae, inactivate lipophilic viruses)
1. Nitrofurazone (Furacin)
2. Oxychlorosene sodium (Chlorpactin)

ANTIPROTOZOAL DRUGS

A. **Antimalarials (Treatment and Prophylaxis)**
  I. **Alkaloids of Cinchona bark**: Quinine and its salts
   1. Quinine sulphate
   2. Quinine bisulphate
   3. Quinine hydrochloride
   4. Quinine dihydrochloride
  II. **Acridine Derivatives**: Mepacrine hydrochloride
  III. **4-Aminoquinoline Derivatives**:
   1. Amodiaquine
   2. Chloroquine phosphate
   3. Chloroquine sulphate
   4. Hydroxychloroquine sulphate
  IV. **8-Aminoquinoline Derivatives**: Primaquine phosphate
  V. **Biguanides**: Proguaril hydrochloride
  VI. **Diaminopyrimidine**: Pyrimethamine
  VII. **Sulphonamides**:
   1. Sulphadoxine (for plasmodium falciparum infection)
   2. Fansidar (Pyrimethamine+Sulpahdoxine)
   3. Maloprim (Pyrimethamine+Dapsone)-for prophylaxis
   4. Cotrimoxazole (Chloroquine resistant malaria)
  VIII. **Inhibitors of Folate Synthesis**
   1. Pyrimethamine
   2. Proguanil (its triazine metabolite, cycloguanil is active)
   3. Fansidar(Sulfadoxine 500mg+Pyrimethamine25mg)per tablet
  IX. **Antibiotics**
   1. Tetracycline
   2. Doxycycline
   3. Clindamycin

X. **Atovaquone** (a hydroxynaphthoquinone)
　　Malarone (Atovaquone250mg+Proguanil100mg)
XI. **Halofantrine & Lumefantrine**
XII. **Artemisinin & Its Derivatives**

Drugs for Prevention of Malaria in Travellers

Chloroquine (areas without resistant P falciparum)　　　　500 mg/week
Mefloquine　(areas with chloroquine-resistant P falciparum) 250 mg/week
Doxycyxline (areas with multidrug resistant P falciparum)　100 mg/day
Malarone　　(areas with chloroquine-resistant P falciparum) 1 tab(250mg
　　　　　　atovaquone+100mg proguanil)/day
Primaquine　(Terminal prophylaxis of P vivax & P ovale)　26.3mg(15mg
　　　　　　base) daily for 14 days after travel.

B. Amoebicides (Antiamoebic Drugs)

I. All types of Amoebiasis (Intestinal and extra-intestinal)
　　　Metronidazole
　　　Tinidazole
　　　Niridazole
II. Mainly Acting in Intestinal Lumen
　a. Diloxanide furoate
　　　　i. Etofamide
　　　　ii. Clefamide
　　　　ii. Teclozen
　b. Chioquinol (iodochlorhydroxyquin)
　　　　i. Diiodhydroxyquin
　　　　ii. Clinifon
　　　　iii. Broxyquinolone
　c. Acetarsol
　　　　i. Carbarsone
　　　　ii. Glycobiarsol
　d. Tetracycline
　　　　Paromomycin
III. Drugs acting as Tissue Amoebicides
　a. Acting principally in the intestinal wall
　　　　i. Emetine

       ii. Dehydroemetine
       iii. Emetine Bismuth iodide
  b. Acting in the liver: Chloroquine
C. Drug Treatment for Trichomoniasis (Trichomonacides)
   1. Drugs used orally
       i. Metronidazole
       ii. Tinidazole
       iii. Nimorazole
   2. Drugs used locally as pessaries
       i. Acetarsol
       ii. Clioquinol
       iii. Diiodohydroxyquin

D. Drugs for Giardiasis (Antigiardial Drugs)
   1. Metronidazole
   2. Tinidazole
   3. Mepacrine
   4. Diiodhydroxyquin

F. Drugs for Leishmaniasis (Leishmanicides)
   1. Sodium Stibogluconate
   2. Meglumine Antimonate
   3. Urea Stibamine
   4. Pentamidine Isethionate
   5. Hydroxystilbamdine Isethionate

ANTIPROTOZOAL DRUGS

1. Albendazole
2. Atovaquone
3. Atovaquone-proguanil
4. Clindamycin
5. Doxycycline
6. Dehydroemetine
7. Eflornithine
8. Furazolidone
9. Iodoquinol
13. Metronidazole
14. Nifurtimox
15. Paromomycin
16. Pentamidine
17. Pyrimethamine
18. Quinidine gluconate
19. Quinine
20. Sodium stibogluconate
21. Suramin

10. Mefloquine   22. Tetracycline
11. Melarsoprol
12. Trimethoprim-sulfamethoxazole

ANTIFUNGAL AGENTS

I. **According to Mechanism of Action**

    a. **Drugs That Disrupt the Fungal Cell Membrane**
        POLYENES
            1. Amphotericin B
            2. Nystatin
        AZOLES
            1. Imidazoles: Ketoconazole (topical use)
                               Clotrimazole (topical use)
            2. Triazoles: Fluconazole
                               Itraconazole
                               Voriconazole
            3. Allylamines: Terbinafine
                               Naftifine
    b. **Drugs That Inhibit Mitosis:** Griseofulvin
    c. **Drugs That Inhibit DNA Synthesis:** Flucytosine
    d. **Echinocandins** (Inhibits fungal cell wall synthesis):
            Caspofungin

II. **Others**

1. Butaconazole	5. Butenafine	8. Caspofungin
2. Econazole	6. Natamycin	9. Oxiconazole
3. Sulconazole	7. Terconazole	10. Tioconazole
4. Tolnaftate		

ANTIFUNGAL DRUGS

I. ANTIBIOTICS
    1. Nystatin   3. Amphotericin B   5. Condicidin
    2. Natamycin   4. Griseofulvin

II. Imidazoles
  1. Miconazole   3. Clotrimazole   5. Econazole
  2. Isoconazole   4. Ketoconazole
III. Fatty Acids: Zinc Undeceonate
IV. Miscellaneous
  1. Tolnaftate   5. Flucytosine   8. Buclosamide
  2. Chlorphenesin   6. Benzoic acid   9. Salicylic acid
  3. Crystal violet   7. Gentian violet   10. Povidone Iodine
  4. Whitfield's ointment

ANTIFUNGAL DRUGS

1. Systemic Antifungal Drugs For Systemic Infections
  1. Amphotericin B
  2. Flucytosine
  3. Azoles
    i. Ketoconazole
    ii. Itraconazole
    iii. Fluconazole
    iv. Voriconazole
  4. Echinocandins: Caspofungin

2. Systemic Antifungal Drugs for Mucocutaneous Infections
  1. Griseofulvin   2. Terbinafine

3. Topical Antifungal Therapy
  1. Nystatin
  2. Topical azoles: Clotrimazole & Miconazole
  3. Topical allylamines

ANTHELMINTIC DRUGS
(Antihelminthics)

I. Drugs for Hookworm Infestation
  1. Bephenium hydroxynaphthoate
  2. Levamisole
  3. Mebendazole

4. Thiabendazole
5. Pyrental Pamoate
6. Tetrachlorethylene
7. Bitoscanate

II. Drugs for Roundworm Infestation (Ascaricides)
1. Piperazine
2. Bephenium hydroxynaphthoate
3. Mebendazole
4. Thiabendazole
5. Levamisole
6. Pyrental Pamoate
7. Santonin

III. Drugs for Threadworms
1. Piperazine
2. Mebendazole
3. Thiabendazole
4. Pyrental Pamoate
5. Viprynium Embonate

IV. Drugs for Tapeworm Infestation (Taenicides)
1. Niclosamide
2. Mepacrine
3. Dichlorophen
4. Male Fern (Filix Mass)

V. Filaricides (Drugs for Filariasis)
1. Diethylcarbamazine
2. Suramin

VI. Drugs for Schistosomiasis (Schistosomicides)
1. Nirdiaole   2. Stebocaptate
3. Lucanthone   4. Oxamniquine
5. Metrifonate   6. Hycanthone
7. Atibophen
8. Antimony Sodium Tartarte
9. Sodium Antimonyligluconate

ANTHELMINTIC DRUGS

I. ROUNDWORMS (Nematodes)

Ascaris lumbricoides (roundworm)	Albendazole, Pyrantel pamoate, Mebendazole, Piperazine
Trichuris trichura (whipworm)	Albendazole, Mebendazole, Pyrantel pamoate, Oxantel
Necator americanus (hookworm) Ankylostoma duodenale (hookworm)	Albendazole, Pyrantel pamoate, Mebendazole
Enterobius vermicularis (pinworm)	Albendazole, Pyrantel pamoate, Mebendazole
Trichinella spiralis (trichinosis)	Mebendazole+Corticosteroids Albendazole+Corticosteroids
Trichostrongylus species	Pyrantel pamoate, Mebendazole, Albendazole
Cutaneous larva migrans (creeping eruption)	Albendazole, Ivermectin,
Visceral larva migrans	Albendazole, Mebendazole
Angiostrongylus cantonensis	Thiabendazole, Albendazole, Mebendazole
Wuvheraria bancroti (filariasis); Brugia malayi (filariasis); Tropical eosinophilia; Loa loa (Loiasis)	Diethylcarbamazine, Ivermectin
Onchocerca volvulus (onchocerciasis)	Ivermactin
Dracunculus medinensis (guinea worm)	Metronidazole, Thiabendazole, Mebendazole
Capillaria philipinensis (intestinal capillariasis)	Albendazole, Mebendazole, Thiabendazole

II. FLUKES (Trematodes)

Schistosoma haematobium (bilharziasis)	Praziquantel, Metrifonate
Schistosoma mansoni	Praziquantel, Oxamniquine
Schistosoma japonicum	Praziquantel
Clonorchis sinensis(liver fluke); Opisthorchis species	Praziquantel, Albendazole
Paragonimus westermani (lung fluke)	Praziquantel, Bithionol
Fasciola hepatica (sheep liver fluke)	Bithionol, Triclabendazole
Fasciola buski (large intestinal fluke)	Praziquantel, Niclosamide
Heterophyes heterophyes Metagonimus yokogawai (Small intestinal flukes)	Praziquantel, Niclosamide

III. TAPEWORMS (Cestodes)

Taenia saginata (beef tapeworm)	Praziquantel, Niclosamide, Mebendazole
Diphyllobothrium latum (fish tapeworm)	Praziquantel, Niclosamide
Taenia solium (pork tapeworm)	Praziquantel, Niclosamide
Cysticercosis (pork tapeworm larval stage)	Albendazole, Praziquantel
Hymenolepis nana (dwarf tapeworm)	Praziquantel, Niclosamide
Echinococcus granulosus (hydatid disease); Echinococcus multilocularis	

ANTHELMINTIC DRUGS

1. Albendazole
2. Diethylcarbamazine
3. Levamisole
4. Metrifonate
5. Oxamniquine
6. Praziquantel
7. Suramin
8. Oxantel pamoate (Oxantel+pyrantel pamoate)
9. Bithionol
10. Ivermectin
11. Mebendazole
12. Niclosamide
13. Piperazine
14. Pyrantel pamoate
15. Thiabendazole

CANCER CHEMOTHERAPY

A. **CELL CYCLE SPECIFIC**

I. **Anti-Metabolites (Structural Analogs)**
   a. **Folic Acid Antagonist**
      Methotrexate
   b. **Purine Derivatives**
      1. 6 Mercaptopurine
      2. 6 Thioguanine
      3. Azathioprine
      4. Fludarabine
      5. Cladribine
   c. **Pyrimidine Derivatives**
      1. 5-Flourouracil
      2. Cytarabine
      3. Fluoxuridine
      4. Capecitabine
      5. Gemcitabine

II. **Natural Compounds**
   a. **Vinca Alkaloids**
      1. Vincristine
      2. Vinblastine
      3. Vinorelabine
   b. **Epipodophyllotoxins**
      1. Etoposide
      2. Teniposide
   c. **Taxanes**
      1. Docetaxel
      2. Paclitaxel
   d. **Antitumor Antibiotic**
      Bleomycin

B. CELL CYCLE NON-SPECIFIC DRUGS(CCNS)

I. Alkylating Agents
  a. Bis (chlorethyl) amines
    1. Cyclophosphamide
    2. Melphalan
    3. Chlorambucil
    4. Ifosfamide
  b. Alkylsulphones
    1. Busulfan
    2. Tresulfan
  c. Nitrosoureas
    1. Streptozocin
    2. Mustine HCl
    3. Carmustine
    4. Lomustine
    5. Semustine
    6. Estramustine
  d. Aziridines
    1. Thiotepa
    2. Triethylenemalomine
  e. Platinium Derivatives
    1. Cisplatin
    2. Carboplatin
    3. Oxaliplatin
  f. Others (related drugs)
    1. Dacarbazine
    2. Procarbazine
    3. Altretamine

II. Anthracycline
    1. Daunorubicin
    2. Doxorubicin
    3. Epirubicin
    4. Idarubicin
    5. Mitoxantrone

III. Antitumor antibiotics
    1. Dactinomycin   2. Mitomycin

IV. **Camptothecins (Natural Compounds)**
    1. Irinotecan
    2. Topotecan

C. **Hormones & Their Antagonist**
   I. **Male Sex Hormones**
      1. Dromostanolone agonist
      2. Fluoxymesterone
      3. Leuprolide
      4. Flutamide (anti-androgen)
   II. **Female Sex Hormones**
     a. **Estrogens**
       1. Diethylstilbesterol agonist
       2. Eithinylestradiol
       3. Tamoxifen (antiestrogen)
     b. **Progestins**
       1. Medoxyprogesterone
       2. Megesterol
       3. Hydroxyprogesterone
   III. **Adrenocorticosteroids**
      1. Hydrocortisone
      2. Prednisone
   IV. **Gonadotropin – Releasing Hormone**
      1. Goserelin acetate
      2. Leuprolide
   V. **Aromatase Inhibitors**
      1. Aminoglutethimide
      2. Anastrozole
      3. Letrozole
      4. Exemestane

D. **Miscellaneous Anticancer Drugs**
  1. **Enzyme**
      L. Asparaginase
  2. **Substituted Ureas**
      Hydroxyurea
  3. **Imatinib**
  4. **Mitotane**

5. **Retinoic acid derivative**
   Tretinoin
6. **Arsenic Trioxide**
7. **Transtuzumab**
8. **Bone marrow growth factors**
   a. **G-CSF**
      1. Filgrastim
      2. Pegfilgrastim
   b. **GM-CSF**
      Sargramostim
9. **Interferons**
   1. Immune interferon
   2. Lymphoblastic interferon
   3. Fibroblastic interferon

ANTI-CANCER DRUGS

I. **Cytotoxic Drugs**
II. **Corticosteroids**
III. **Sex Hormones**

I. CYTOTOXIC DRUGS

A. **Alkylating Agents**
   1. Cyclophosphamide
   2. Busulphan
   3. Chlorambucil
   4. Melphalan
   5. Mustine Hydrochloride
   6. Thiotepa
   7. Lomustin
   8. Ifosfamide

B. **Antimetabolites**
   1. Folic Acid Analogues
      Methotrexate

2. Pyramidine analogues: Fluorouracil
3. Purine Analogues
   Mercaptopurine
   Aminoglutethimide
   Thioguanine
C. **Vinca Alkaloids**
   1. Vinblastine sulphate 2. Vincristine sulphate
   2. Vindesine sulphate
4. **Cytotoxic Antibiotics**
   1. Actinomycin-D (Dactinomycin)
   2. Bleomycin sulphate
   3. Mitomycin
   4. Mithramycin
   5. Daunarubicin HCl
   6. Doxorubicin
5. **Miscellaneous**
   1. Cisplatin   5. Dacarbazine
   2. Etoposide   6. Hydroxyurea
   3. Procarbazine   7. Tamoxifen
   4. Nafoxidine   8. Asparaginase

II. **CORTICOSTEROIDS**
   1. Prednisolone   3. Prednisone
   2. Prednisone

III. **SEX HORMONES**
1. **Oestrogens**
   i. Stilboestrol
   ii. Fosfestrol Tetrasodium
   iii. Ethanyloestradiol
   iv. Polyoestradiol Phosphate
2. **Progesterogens**
   i. Norethisterone
   ii. Hydroxyprogesterone Hexamoate
   iii. Medroxyprogesteronw Acetate
3. **Androgens and Anabolic Streroids**
   i. Nandrolone Phenylpropionate
   ii. Nandrolone decanoate
   iii. Drostanolone propionate

TUBERCULOSIS

First-line Agents *(in approximate order of preference)*
1. Isoniazid
2. Pyrazinamide
3. Streptomycin
4. Rifampin
5. Ethambutol

Second-line agents
1. Amikacin
2. Aminosalicylate sodium (Sodium P.A.S)
3. Capreomycin
4. Ciprofloxacin
5. Clofazimine
6. Cycloserine
7. Ethionamide
8. Levofloxacin
9. Rifabutin
10. Rifapentine

Drugs active against Atypical Mycobacteria
Erythromycin
Sulfonamides
Tetracycline
Rifampin
Ethambutol
Isoniazid
Combination of Isoniazid, Rifampin, and Ethambutol; Azithromycin 500 mg once daily, or Clarithromycin 500 mg bid, plus Ethambutol 15 mg/kg/d (for disseminated disease)

Recommended Duration Of Therapy For Tuberculosis
1. Isoniazid, Rifampin, Pyrazinamide — 6 months
2. Isoniazid, Rifampin — 9 months
3. Rifampin, Ethambutol, Pyrazinamide — 6 months
4. Rifampin, Ethambutol — 12 months
5. Isoniazid, Ethambutol — 18 months
6. All others — 24 months

IMMUNOPHARMACOLOGY

1. Azathioprine
2. Basiliximab (Simulect)
3. Bacillus Calmettes-Guerin, BCG live (Thoracys, Tice)
4. Cyclophosphamide (Cytoxan, Neosar)
5. Cyclosporine (Sandimmune, Neoral, SangCya)
6. Daclizumab (Zenapax)
7. Entanercept (Enbrel)
8. Glatiramer (Copaxone)
9. Immune Globulin 10.
10. Intravenous (IGIV, Gamimmune, Gammagard, Polygam)
11. Infliximab (Remicade)
12. Interferon alpha-2a (Roferon) -2b(Interon)
13. Interferon beta-1b (Betaseron)
14. Interferon gamma-1b (Actimmune)
15. Interleukin-2, IL-2, Aldesleukin (Prolukin)
16. Leflunomide (Arava)
17. Levamisole (Ergamisol)
18. Lymphocyte immune globulin (Atgam)
19. Methylprednisolone sodium succinate (Solu-Medrol)
20. Muromonab-CD3 (Orthoclone OKT3)
21. Mycophenolate mofetil (CellCept)
22. Pegademase Bovine (Adegen)
23. Prednisone
24. Rh (D)Immune Globulin Mini-dose(HypRho-D,MICRhoGAM)
25. Rituximab (Rituxan)
26. Sirolimus (Rapamune)
27. Tacrolimus (Prograf)
28. Thalidomide (Thalomid)
29. Trastuzumab (Herceptin)

IMMUNOMODULANTS

A. **IMMUNOSUPRESSIVE AGENTS**
  I. **Adrenocortical Steroid**
   1. Prednisone
   2. Prednisolone
  II. **Calcineurin Inhibitors**
   1. Cyclosporin
   2. Tacrolimus
  III. **Antiproliferative and Antimetabolites**
   1. Azathioprine
   2. Mercaptopurine
   3. Methotrexate
   4. Cyclophosphamide
   5. Mycophenolate Mofetil
   6. Sirolimus
  IV. **Antibody Reagents**
   1. Antithymocyte Antibodies
   2. Antilymphocyte Antibodies
   3. Immunoglobulins
   4. Monoclonal Antibodies
        i. Trastuzumab   ii. Rituximab
        iii. Daclizumab   iv. Abciximab
        v. Palvizumab

B. **IMMUNOSTIMULANTS**
  I. **Natural adjuvant**
        BCG
  II. **Synthetic Agents**
        Levamisole
        Isoprinosine
  III. **Cytokines**
        Interferon alpha
        GM – CSF
        G-CSF
        Interleukin

ACTIVE IMMUNISATION AGENTS

Diphtheria-tetanus-acellular pertussis (Toxoid+inactivated bacteria)	IM
Haemophilus influenzae type b conjugate (Bacterial polysaccharide)	IM
Hepatitis A (Inactivated virus)	IM
Hepatitis B (Inactivated viral antigen, recombinant)	IM, SC
Influenza (Inactivated virus or viral components)	IM
Measles (Live virus)	SC
Measles-mumps-rubella (MMR) (Live virus)	SC
Meningococcal vaccine (Bacterial polysaccharides)	SC
Mumps (Live virus)	SC
Pneumococcal vaccine (Bacterial polysaccharides-23 serotypes)	IM, SC
Poliovirus vaccine, inactivated (IPV) (Inactivated viruses-3 serotypes)	SC
Rabies (Inactivated virus)	IM, ID
Rubella (Live virus)	SC
Tetanus-diphtheria (TD or DT) (Toxoid)	IM
Typhoid, Ty 21 an oral (Live bacteria)	Oral
Typhoid, Vi capsular polysaccharide (Bacterial polysaccaharide)	IM
Varicella (Live virus)	SC
Yellow fever (Live virus)	SC

TOXICOLOGY

HEAVY METAL INTOXICATION & CHELATORS

Heavy Metals Intoxication	Chelators
Iron salts	Deferoxamine (Desferal)
Arsenic, Gold, Mercury	Dimercaprol (BAL in oil)
Copper, lead and gold	Penicillamine (Cuprimine, Depen)
Lead	Calcium disodium ethylenediamine tetraacetate (Ca EDTA) Dimercaprol
Arsenic	Unithiol, Dimercaprol
Mercury	Metal chelators, N-Acetylpenicillamine Dimercaprol Succimer Unithiol

POISONS AND THEIR ANTIDOTES

Toxin	Antidotes
Acetaminophen	N-Acetylcystine
Anticholinesterases	Atropine Physostigmine
Benzodiazepines	Flumazenil
Beta blockers	Glucagon
Calcium channel blockers	Calcium
Digitalis glycosides	Digoxin-specific antibody fragments
Iron salts	Deferoxamine (Deferal)
Isoniazid, Hydrazine	Pyridoxone (Vit. B 6)
Opiates	Naloxone
Organophosphates or insecticides	Atropine Pralidoxine
Methanol or Ethylene glycol	Ethanol Fomepizole (Antizol)
Tricyclic antidepressants	Bicarbonate

SPECIAL TOPICS

ANTI-LEPROSY DRUGS

1. Dapsone (diaminodiphenylsulfone)
2. Colfazimine
3. Mioacetazone
4. Rifampicin
5. Thiambutosine
6. Ditophal

VENEREAL DISEASES

I. Drugs for Gonorrhoea

1. Proacine Penicillin — 1-2 g IM Injection
2. Ampicillin — 2-3.5 g orally
3. Spectinomycin — 2 g IM Injection for males
   4 g IM Injection for females
4. Cotrimoxazole — 4 tablets 12 hourly for 2 days
5. Acrosoxacin — 300 mg as a single dose

II. Drugs for Syphilis

Primary and Secondary Syphilis
1. Procaine Penicillin, 600 mg IM injection for 10 days
2. Benzathine Penicillin 45mg/Kg IM injection for 3 weeks

Tertiary Syphilis
Procaine Penicillin, 600 mg IM injection for 3 weeks

Congenital Syphilis
1. Procaine Penicillin, 45 mg IM injection for 10 days
2. Tetracycline 3 g daily for 3 weeks

VACCINES AND SERA
(Immunological Products)

1. Anthrax vaccine
2. Cholera vaccine
3. Diphtheria vaccine
4. Diphtheria and Tetanus vaccine
5. Diphtheria, Tetanus and Pertussis vaccine (Trivax-AD)
6. Diphtheria vaccine TAF (Toxoid-antitoxin floccules)
7. Hepatitis B Vaccine
8. Influenza Vaccine
9. Measles Vaccine
10. Mumps vaccine
11. Poliomyelitis vaccine (Oral)
12. Poliomyelitis vaccine (Killed or inactivated) (Injectable)
13. Rabies vaccine
14. Rubella vaccine
15. Smallpox vaccine

IMMUNOGLOBULINS

1. Human Normal Immunoglobulins (HNIG, German Globulin)
2. Antirabies immunoglobulin
3. Antitetanus immunoglobulin (HTIG)
4. Antivaccinia immunoglobulin

VARICES HEMORRHAGE

1. Somatostatin
2. Octreotide
3. Vasopressin
4. Terlipressin
5. Beta Receptor Blocking Drugs

ANTIDIARRHEAL DRUGS

I. Prolong Intestinal Transit Time by Reducing Motility
   a. Naturally Occuring Opium Alkaloids
      1. Codeine phosphate
      2. Morphine
      3. Opium Tincture
   b. Synthetic Opiate Compounds
      1. Diphenoxylate
      2. Loperamide
   c. Anticholinergics
      1. Belladona   3. Atropine
      2. Propantheline   4. Dicyclomine HCl

II. Drugs that Increase Bulk of Intestinal Contents
      1. Methylcellulose   4. Activated Attapulgite
      2. Light Kaolin   5. Sterculia
      3. Ispaghula Husk

III. Miscellaneous
      1. Peppermint Oil
      2. Vegetable Astringents

SELECTED ANTIDIARRHEAL DRUGS
      1. Bismuth subsalicylate
      2. Difenoxin
      3. Difenoxylate
      4. Kaolin+pectin (Kaopectate)
      5. Loperamide
      6. Paregoric

DIGESTANTS
      1. Pancreatin
      2. Pepsin and Papain
      3. Diastase

DIGESTIVE ENZYMES
      1. Pancrelipase
      2. Pancreatin

IRRITABLE BOWEL SYNDROME (IBS)

1. **Antidiarrhoeal Agents**: Loperamide
2. **Osmotic Laxatives**: Milk of magnesia
3. **Tricyclic Antidepressants**
       Amitryptaline   10-25 mg/day
       Desipramine: 10-25 mg/day
4. **Antispasmodics (Anticholinergics)**
   1. Dicyclomine
   2. Hyoscyamine
5. **Serotonin 5-HT3 Receptor Antagonists**
   1. Alosetron
   2. Ondansetron
   3. Ganisetron
   4. Dolasetron

INFLAMMATORY BOWEL DISEASES (IBD)
(Ulcerative Colitis & Crohn's Disease)

1. **Aminosalicylates** (5-aminosalicylic acid compounds:5-ASA)
   Azo compounds
       i. Sulfasalazine
       ii. Balsalazide
       iii. Olsalazine
   Mesalamine compounds
       i. Pentasa
       ii. Asacol (Rectally-Rowasa; Suppository-Canasa)
2. **Glucocorticoids**
       i. Prednisolone
       ii. Budesonide (Entocort)
3. **Purine Analogs (Purine antimetabolites)**
       i. Azathioprine
       ii. 6-Mercaptopurine
4. **Methotrexate (Antimetabolite)**
       Anti-TNF-Alpha Therapy: Infliximab

APPETITE SUPPRESSANTS

I. Bulk Forming Drugs
   Methylcellulose and Sterculia

II. Centrally Acting Appetite Suppressants
   1. Fenfluramine HCl
   2. Mazindol
   3. Phenmetrazine HCl
   4. Methamphetamine
   5. Diethylpropin
   6. Phentermine HCl
   7. Amphetamine

ANTIEMETICS

A. PHENOTHIAZINES
   Centrally acting (acting on CTZ)
   1. Chlorpromazine
   2. Prochlorperazine
   3. Perfenazine
   4. Thiethylperazine

   Centrally & peripherally acting (Chemoreceptor trigger zone, CTZ & GIT)
   1. Domperidone
   2. Metoclopramide

B. ANTIHISTAMINE (H1 receptor antagonist)
   1. Cyclizine
   2. Promethazine
   3. Cinarizine
   4. Dimenhydrinate

C. 5-HT3 SEROTONIN RECEPTOR ANTAGONIST
   1. Ondansetron
   2. Granisetron
   3. Dolasetron
   4. Tropisetron

D. SUBSTITUTED BENZAMIDES: Metocopramide

E. ANTIMUSCARINIC DRUGS
   Hyoscine

F. CANNABINOID RECEPTOR BLOCKERS
   (Marijuana derivatives): Dronabinol

G. **MISCELLANEOUS**
    1. Benzodiazepines: Lorazepam
    2. Corticosteroids: Dexamethasone

ANTIEMETICS

A. **Depressants of Chemoreceptor trigger zone (CTZ) & Vomiting Centre**
    1. **Anticholinergic Drugs**: Hyoscine (Scopolamine)
    2. **Antihistamines**
        1. Cyclizine
        2. Hydroxyzine
        3. Meclozine
        4. Promethazine theoclate
    3. **Tranquillizers**
       Phenothiazines
        1. Chlorpromazine
        2. Trifluoperazine
        3. Perfenazine
        4. Prochlorperazine maleate
        5. Prochlorperazine mesylate
        6. Thiethylperazine
    4. **Accelerator of Gastric Emptying:** Metoclopramide

B. **Drugs Acting By Removing Spasm**
    i. **Relieving Myogenic Spasm**
       Volatile oils, Spirits, Camphor, Menthol, Chloroform
    ii. **Relieving Neurogenic Spasm**: Anticholinergics
       Atropine, Hyoscine, Hyoscyamine, Probanthine
    iii. **Locally Acting**
       i. **Demulcents, Adsorbents and Mild Astringents**
          1. Gum acacia
          2. Kaolin
          3. Bismuth carbonate
          4. Mucilage of Tragacanth
          5. Alumium hydroxide
       ii. **Local Anaesthetics**
          1. Chlorobutanes
          2. Oxethazaine

EMETICS

1. *Centrally Acting*: Apomorphine
2. *Reflexly Acting:* Ipecac, Tar Tar Emetic
3. *Locally Acting:* Alum, Copper Sulphate, Zinc Sulphate, Sodium Chloride

BITTERS

1. *Simple bitters*: Gentian, Quassia, Calumba
2. *Astringent bitters*: Cusparia, Cascarilla
3. *Aromatic bitters*: Orange peel, Lemon peel
4. *Alkaloidal bitters*:
    Cinchona bark (contains Quinine)
    Nux vomica (contains Strychnine)

ANTITUSSIVES

I. CENTRAL ANTITUSSIVES

   A. Narcotic Antitussives

      a. Relatively Less Addicting Drugs
        1. Codeine Phosphate
        2. Dihydrocodeine Tartrate
        3. Pholcodine
      b. Addicting Drugs
        1. Camphoarated Opium Tincture
        2. Concentrated Camphoarated Opium Tincture
        3. Morphine sulphate
        4. Methadone HCl
        5. Diamorphine HCl
        6. Dihydromorphine
        7. Ethylmorphine
        8. Isoeminile citrate

   B. Non-Narcotic (Non-addicting) Antitussives

      a. Opiate Derivatives
        1. Dextromethorphan HBr
        2. Noscapine
        3. Levopropoxyphene Napsylate

b. **Non-opiate Synthetic Derivatives**
   1. Carbetapentane
   2. Chlorphedianol
   3. Caramiphen ethane disulphonate
   4. Benzonatate
   5. Diphenhydramine
II. **PERIPHERAL ANTITUSSIVES**

   a. **Demulcents**: Liquorice (Glycerrhiza)
   b. **Steam Inhalation**: Benzoin
   c. **Drugs with Local Anaesthetic Activity**
      Benzonatate (it has both central and peripheral activity)
   d. **Miscellaneous**: Dropropizine

CARBONIC ANHYDRASE INHIBITORS

1. **Systemic**

   1. Acetazolamide (the prototype agent)
   2. Dichlorphenamide
   3. Methazolamide

2. **Local (instilled in eye)**

   1. Dorzolamide
   2. Brinzolamide

EXPECTORANTS/ MUCOLYTIC

EXPECTORANTS

Drugs Acting Reflexly
1. Ipecacuanha
2. Ammonium chloride
3. Ammonium bicarbonate
4. Senega
5. Guaiphenasin
6. Cocillana
7. Squill
8. Terpin hydrate

MUCOLYTIC

I. Inhalational Mucolytics
   1. Acetylcysteine
   2. Tyloxapol

II. Oral Mucolytics
   1. Acetylcysteine
   2. Bromhexine
   3. Carbocisteine
   4. Methylcysteine

RESPIRATORY STIMULANTS (Analeptics)

1. Nikethamide
2. Ethamivan
3. Amiphenazole
4. Pentetrazol
5. Aromatic spirit of ammonia
6. Doxapram
7. Lobeline
8. Bemegride
9. Picrotoxin
10. Helium gas

DRUGS ACTING ON GALL BLADDER

1. **Cholagogues**:(Stimulate the flow of bile from gall bladder to duodenum)
   Magnesium sulphate
2. **Choleretics**: (Stimulate liver cells to secrete bile)

   Natural Bile Acids and their Derivatives
   Chenodeoxycholic acid (Chendol, Chenofolk)
   Ursodeoxycholic acid (Destilit, Ursofalk)
   Dehydrocholic acid

GALLSTONES DISSOLVING AGENTS

1. Monoctanoin (Moctanin)
2. Ursodiol (Actigal, Urso)

OPEN ANGLE GLAUCOMA

I. **Drugs Administered Topically**
    (a) **Parasympathomimetics**
        Pilocarpine HCl
        Pilocarpine Nitrate
        Carbachol
    (b) **Anticholinesterases**
        Physostigmine sulphate
        Echothiophate
        Demecarium
    (c) **Adrenergic Neurone Blocking Drugs**
        Guanethidine
    (d) **Sympathomimetics**: Adrenaline, Dipivefrin
    (e) **Beta Adrenergic Blocking Agents**
        1. Timolol
        2. Betaxolol
        3. Carteolol
        4. Levobunolol (Betagan liquifilm)
        5. Metipranolol (Optipranolol)

II. **Drugs Administered Systemically**

    (a) **Carbonic Anhydrase Inhibitors**
        1. Acetazolamide
        2. Dichlorphenamide

    (b) **Osmotic Agents**
        1. Glycerol
        2. Isosorbide
        3. Mannitol
        4. Urea

GASTROINTESTINAL TRACT

Anti-Inflammatory (Selected Drugs) For GIT Diseases

1. Hydrocortisone
2. Methylprednisolone
3. Sulfasalazine
4. Balsalazide
5. Mesalamine
6. Olsalazine
7. Infliximab
8. Budesonide

PEPTIC ULCER/H.PYLORI

A. **DRUGS THAT REDUCE ACID/PEPSIN ACTIVITY**

1. **Gastric Antacids**
   a. **Systemic**
      Sodium Bicarbonate
   b. **Non- Systemic**
      i. **Physico-Chemically Acting**
         Aluminium Hydroxide
         Aluminium Phosphate
         Magnesium Trisilicate
      ii. **Chemically Acting**
         Magnesium Oxide
         Magnesium Hydroxide
         Magnesium Carbonate
         Calcium Carbonate
         Bismuth
2. **H2 Receptor Anatgonists**
   1. Cimetidine
   2. Ranitidine
   3. Famotidine
   4. Nizatidine
3. **Proton Pump Inhibitors(Benzimidazole Derivatives)**
   1. Omeprazole
   2. Lansoprazole
   3. Rabeprazole
   4. Esomeprazole
   5. Pantoprazole

    4. M 1 Selective Anticholinergic Drug
        Pirenzepine
    5. Somatostatin Analog
        Octreotide
B. MUCOSAL PROTECTIVE AGENTS
    1. Sulfated Sucrose Derivative
        Sucralfate
    2. Colloidal Bismuth Compounds
        Bismuth subcitrate
    3. Prostaglandin Derivative
        Misoprostol
    4. Liquorice Derivative
        Carbenoxolone
C. MISCELLANEOUS
    1. Metoclopramide (prokinetic)
    2. Simethicone (antifoaming deflatulant)
    3. Oxethazine (local anaesthetic, present in Mucaine)
D. DRUGS FOR ERADICATION OF H. PYLORI
    Metronidazole, Tetracycline / Amoxicillin & Bismuth subcitrate
    OR
    Metronidazole, Amoxicillin / Clarithromycin & Omeprazole
    OR
    Omeprazole & Clarithromycin
    OR
    Omeprazole & Amoxicillin
    OR
    Ranitidine, Bismuth subcitrate & one Antibiotic

PEPTIC ULCER
(Acid-Peptic Disease)

1. ANTACIDS
    a. Systemic: Sodium bicarbonate
    b. Non-Systemic
        Aluminium salts:
            Aluminium Hydroxide Gel
            Aluminium Glycinate
            Aluminium Phosphate

ii. *Magnesium salts*
  Magnesium Trisilicate
  Magnesium Hydroxide
  Magnesium Oxide
  Magnesium Carbonate
  iii. *Calcium salts*: Calcium Carbonate
  iv. *Bismuth salts*: Bismuth Subcarbonate
  V. *Combination*
  Aluminium Hydroxide, Magnesium Hydroxide
  (Mylanta, Gaviscon, Gelucil, Maalox)
2. **H-2 RECEPTOR ANTAGONISTS** *(H-2 Histamine Receptor Blockers)*
   1. Cimetidine
   2. Ranitidine
   3. Famotidine
   4. Nizatidine
2. **PROTON PUMP INHIBITORS (PPI)**
   1. Omeprazole
   2. Lansoprazole
   3. Rabeprazole
   4. Pantoprazole
   5. Esomeprazole
4. **ANTICHOLINERGIC DRUGS**
   a. Natural: *Belladona alkaloids, extract or tincture*
   1. Atropine
   2. L-Hyoscyamine
   b. Semisynthetic: Hyoscine butylbromide
   c. Synthetic
   i. *Tertiary Amines*
   1. Dicyclomine
   2. Piperodolate
   ii. *Quaternary Ammonium Compounds*
   1. Propantheline
   2. Poldine
   3. Pipenzolate
   d. Selective Anticholinergics: Pirenzepine

5. SULPHATED SUCROSE COMPLEX: Sucralfate
6. LIQUORICE DERIVATIVES
      1. Carbenoxolone (Biogastrone, Duogastrone)
      2. Deglycyrrhizinised liquorice
7. BISMUTH CHELATE: Tripotassium dicitrobismuthate (de-Nol)
8. MUCOSAL PROTECTIVE AGENTS
      1. Sucralfate
      2. Prostaglandin analogs
      3. Colloidal bismuth compounds
      4. Misoprostol
9. MISCELLANEOUS
      1. Metoclopramide
      2. Oxethazaine
      3. Simethicone
      4. Proglumide
      5. Prostaglandins

SIALOGOGUES

1. Reflexly Acting
i. Acting within the mouth
    By mechanical Means: Chewing gums
    By Chemical Means
        Bitter Stomachics
        Dilute Acids (Citric & Tartaric acids)
        Dilute Alcohols
        Acid Juices (Lemon & Orange Juices)
        Volatile Oils
        Pungent Salts
        Ether
ii. Acting via Gastric Nerve Endings: *Small doses of emetics*
2. Acting on Salivary Mechanism
  i. Parasympathomimetics
  ii. Stimulans of Autonomic Ganglia (due to parasympathetic stimulation)
  iii. Direct Stimulants of acini (during excretion through salivary glands):
      Iodides & Mercurials

ANTISIALOGOGUES

1. **Drugs which Allay Irritation of Mouth**
Demulsants and astringent mouth gargle of borax, boric acid, alum
2. **Parasympatholytics**
   Antimuscarinics i.e., atropine-like drugs
3. **Ganglion Blocking Drugs** (due to parasympathetic blockade)
   1. Pentolinium
   2. Mecamylamine
4. **Centrally acting Drugs**: Opium and its derivatives

MOTILITY DISORDERS & SELECTED ANTIEMETICS

1. Cisapride
2. Dronabinol
3. Metoclopramide
4. Prochlorperazine
5. Tegaserod
6. Dolasetron
7. Granisetron
8. Ondansetron
9. Alosetron

PURGATIVES
(According to Mechanism of Action)

1. **Bulk-forming Purgatives**
   i. Bran
   ii. Psyllium Husk
   iii. Calcium Polycarbophil
   iv. Ispaghula Husk
   v. Cellulose
2. **Stimulant purgatives**
   i. Castor Oil
   i. Diphenylmethane derivative
   iii. Bisacodyl
   iv. Anthraquinone derivative
      a. Senna
      b. Rhubarb

3. **Fecal Softeners (Stool Surfactant Agents)**
   i. Glycerin
   ii. Mineral oil (e.g liquid paraffin)
4. **Osmotic Laxatives**
   i. Magnesium Sulphate
   ii. Lactulose
   iii. Mannitol

PURGATIVES

I. According to Intensity of Action
Laxative, Purgative and Drastic in the order of increasing potency

II. Site of Action
   a. Small gut only: Castor oil, irritant resins
   b. Large gut only
      Anthracine purgatives
      Bisacodyl
      Phenolphthalein
   c. Large and small: Saline purgatives and lubricants

III. Mechanism of Action
   A. Stimulant Purgatives   **B. Bulk-forming drugs**
   C. Faecal softeners   **D. Miscellaneous drugs**

A. STIMULANT PURGATIVES (Cathartics)

I. Drugs which act mainly on large intestine
   a. Bisacodyl
   b. Anthraquinone Derivatives
         1. Senna   4. Cascara sagrada
         2. Rheubarb   5. Aloes
         3. Danthron

ii. Drugs which act mainly on small intestine
   a. Oils: Castor oil
   b. Resins: Podophyllym, Jalap

B. BULK-FORMING DRUGS

i. Colloidal purgatives

    a. **Natural Plant Products**
    1. Methylcellulose   4. Psyllium   6. Bran
    2. Ispaghula   5. Sterculia   7. Agar-Agar
    3. Frangula
    b. **Synthetic Fibers**   Polycarbophil

ii. Osmotic purgatives

    Saline purgatives
      i. Magnesium sulphate   Magnesium hydroxide
         Magnesium oxide   Magnesium carbonate
         Sodium sulphate   Sodium potassium tartrate
      ii. Lactulose

C. FAECAL SOFTENERS

a. Lubricants: Liquid paraffin and vegetable oils
b. Dioctyl sodium sulphosuccinate

D. MISCELLANEOUS DRUGS

Drastic action: Colocynth, Jalap, Podophyllum
Parasympathomimetics
    1. Bethanichol   2. Neostigmine
    3. Distigmine   4. Pyridostigmine

SELECTED LAXATIVE DRUGS

a. Bisacodyl   g. Cascara sagrada   l. Castor oil
b. Docusate   h. Glycerin liquid   m. Glycerin suppository
c. Lactulose   j. Methylcellulose   n. Mineral oil
d. Polycarbophil k. Psyllium   o. Senna
e. Magnesium hydroxide (Milk of magnesia, Epsom Salt)
f. Polyethylene glycol electrolyte solution

MISCELLANEOUS

SPECIAL ASPECTS OF PERI-NATAL AND PAEDIATRIC PHARMACOLOGY

Drugs with Significant Adverse Effects on Fetus

Drug	Trimester	Effect
ACE inhibitors	All, esp. 2nd & 3rd	Renal damage
Aminopterin	1st	Multiple gross anomalies
Amphetamines	All	Abnormal developmental patterns, decreased school performance
Androgens	2nd & 3rd	Masculinization of female fetus
Antidepressants, Tricylic	3rd	Neonatal withdrawal symptoms with clomipramine, desipramine, imipramine
Barbiturates	All	Chronic use can lead to neonatal dependence
Busulfan	All	Congenital malformation, low birth weight
Carbamazepine	1st	Neural tube defects
Chlorpropamide	All	Prolonged symptomatic neonatal hypoglycemia
Clomipramine	3rd	Neonatal lethargy, hypotonia, cyanosis, hypothermia
Cocaine	All	Spontaneous abortion, abruptio placentae, premature labor; neonatal cerebral infarction, abnormal development, decreased school performance
Cyclophosphamide	1st	Congenital malformations
Cytarabine	1st & 2nd	Congenital malformations
Diazepam	All	Chronic use may lead to neonatal dependence and risk for oral cleft
Diethylstilbestrol	All	Vaginal adenosis, clear cell vaginal adenocarcinoma

Ethanol	All	Fetal alcohol syndrome, alcohol-related neurodevelopmental defects
Etritinate	All	Multiple congenital malformations
Heroin	All	Neonatal dependence
Iodide	All	Congenital goiter, hypothyroidism
Isotretinoin	All	CNS, face, ear malformation
Lithium	1st	Ebstein's anomaly
Methadone	All	Neonatal dependence
Methotrexate	1st	Multiple congenital malformations
Methylthiouracil	All	Hypothyroidism
Metronidazole	1st	May be mutagenic
Organic solvents	1st	Multiple malformations
Misoprostol	1st	Mobius sequence
Penicillamine	1st	Cutis laxa, other congenital malformations
Phencyclidine	All	Abnormal neurologic examination, poor suck reflex and feeding
Phenytoin	All	Featl hydantoin syndrome
Propylthiouracil	All	Congenital goiter
Streptomycin	All	Eighth nerve toxicity
Smoking, tobacco	All	Intrauterine growth retardation, prematurity; sudden infant death syndrome; perinatal complications
Tamoxifen	All	Risk of spontaneous abortion, fetal damage
Tetracycline	All	Discoloration and defects of teeth and altered bone growth
Thalidomide	1st	Phocomelia (shortened or absent long bones of the limbs) and many internal malformations
Trimethadone	All	Multiple congenital anomalies
Valproic acid	All	Neural tube defects

DRUGS USED DURING LACTATION AND THEIR EFFECTS ON THE NURSING INFANT

Drug	Effect	Comments
Ampicillin	Minimal	Diarrhea or allergic sensitization
Aspirin	Minimal	Significant amount in breast milk with high doses
Caffeine	Minimal	In breast milk it is 1% of that in maternal blood
Chloral hydrate	Significant	Drowsiness
Chloramphenicol	Significant	Bone marrow suppression; stop breast feeding while using chloramphenicol
Chlorothiazide	Minimal	No adverse effects reported
Chlorpromazine	Minimal	Appears insignificant
Codeine	Minimal	No adverse effects reported
Diazepam	Significant	Sedation; may accumulate in newborn
Dicumoral	Minimal	No adverse effects; follow prothrombin time
Digoxin	Minimal	Insignificant quantities in breast milk
Ethanol	Moderate	Alcohol effects in infant
Heroin	Significant	Can prolong neonatal narcotic dependence
Iodine: radioactive	Significant	Thyroid suppression in infants
Isoniazid	Minimal	Pyridoxine deficiency in infant
Kanamycin	Minimal	No adverse effects reported
Lithium	Significant	Nursing only if levels can be measured
Methadone	Significant	(See heroin) Under close physician can be continued. Signs of opiate withdrawal in the infant may occur if mother stops taking methadone or stops breast feeding abruptly
Oral contraceptives	Minimal	May suppress lactation in high doses
Penicillin	Minimal	Very low concentration in breast milk
Phenobarbital	Moderate	Hypnotic doses cause sedation in infant
Phenytoin	Moderate	No adverse effects
Prednisone	Moderate	Doses more than 15mg be avoided
Propranolol	Minimal	Very small amounts enter breast milk
Propylthiouracil	Significant	Can suppress thyroid function in infant
Spironolactone	Minimal	Very small amounts enter breast milk

Tetracycline	Moderate	Permanent staining of developing teeth in infant. Should not be used.
Theophylline	Moderate	Not likely to produce significant effects
Thyroxine	Minimal	No adverse effects in therapeutic doses
Tolbutamide	Minimal	Low concentration in breast milk
Warfarin	Minimal	Very small quantities found in milk

ERECTILE DYSFUNCTION (ED)

I. Oral Phosphodiesterase Inhibtors/PDE-5 Inhibitors (First line therapy)
    1. Sildenafil
    2. Tadalafil
    3. Vardenafil

II. Previous Therapies
    1. Penile implants
    2. Intrapenile injections of alprostadil
    3. Intraurethral suppositories of alprostadil

OSTEOPOROSIS

I. Bisphosphanates (The Analogs of Pyrophosphate)

    1. Etidronate
    2. Risedronate
    3. Alendronate (also used for prevention of osteoporosis)
    4. Pamidronate
    5. Ibandronate

II. Teriparatide: A recombinant segment of human parathyroid hormine

III. Selected Estrogen-receptor Modulators (SERMs): Raloxifene

IV. Calcitonin

OBESITY

1. Phentermine
2. Sibutramine
3. Ortistat

DERMATOLOGIC PHARMACOLOGY

A. **Topical Antifungal Preparations**
 1. Topical azole derivatives
    Imidazoles
       Clotrimazole
       Econazole
       Ketoconazole
       Miconazole
       Oxiconazole
       Sulconazole
       Clotrimazole-betamethasone dipropionate
 2. Ciclopirex Olamine
 3. Naftifine
 4. Terbinafine
 5. Butinafine hydrochoride
 6. Tolnaftate
 7. Nystatin & Amphotericin B

B. **Oral Antifungal Agents**
 1. Griseofulvin
 2. Oral azole derivatives
    Fluconazole
    Itraconazole
    Ketoconazole
 3. Terbinafine

C. **Topical Antiviral Agents**
 1. Acyclovir
 2. Penciclovir
 3. Valacyclovir
 4. Famciclovir

D. Immunomodulators
1. Imiquimod
2. Tacrolimus & Pimecrolimus

E. Ectoparasiticides
1. Lindane (Hexachlorcyclohexane)
2. Sulfur
3. Malathion
4. Crotamiton
5. Permethrin

F. Agents affecting Pigmentation
1. Hydroquinone
2. Trioxsalen
3. Monobenzone
4. Methoxsalen

G. Sunscreens
1. Opaque Maretials or sunshades (that reflect light): Titanium dioxide
2. P-aminobenzoic acid (PABA) & its esters
3. Benzophenones
    Oxybenzone
    Dioxybenzone
    Sulisobenzone
4. Dibenzoylmethanes
    Parsol
    Eusolex

H. Acne Preparations
1. Retinoic acid & Derivatives
    Adaplene (Diferin)
    Tazarotene (Tazorac)
2. Isotretinoin (Accutane)
3. Benzoyl Peroxide
    Benzoyl peroxide+Eryhthrocin (Benzamycin)
    Benzoyl peroxide+Clindamycin (BenzaClin)
4. Azelaic Acid (Azelex)

J. Drugs for Psoriasis
    1. Acitretin (Soriatane)   2. Tazarotene (Tazorac)
    3. Calcipotriene (Dovonex)

K. Anti-Inflammatory Agents
    1. Topical Corticosteroids
    2. Alefacept (Amevive)
    3. Tar compounds

L. Keratolytic and Destructive Agents
    1. Salicylic acid
    2. Propylene glycol
    3. Urea
    4. Podophyllum resin & Podofilox
    5. Fluorouracil
    6. Aminolevulinic acid

M. Antipruritic Agents
    1. Doxepin (Zonalon)
    2. Pramoxine

N. Trichogenic & Antitrichogenic Agents
    1. Minoxidil, topical (Rogaine)
    2. Finasteride (Propecia)
    3. Eflornithine (Vaniqa)

O. Antiseborrhea Agents
    1. Betamethasone valerate foam (Luxiq)
    2. Chloroxine shampoo (Capitrol)
    3. Coal tar shampoo (Lonil-T, Theraplex-T,T-Gel)
    4. Flucinilone acetonide shampoo (FS Shampoo)
    5. Ketoconazole shampoo (Nizoral)
    6. Selenium sulfide shampoo (Selsun, Exsel)
    7. Zinc pyrithione shampoo (DHS-zinc, Theraplex-Z)

P. Anti-neoplastic Agents: Aletretinoin (Panretin)

Agents That Enhance Drug Metabolism in Humans

Inducer	Drug whose metabolism is enhanced
Benzo (a)pyrene	Theophylline
Chlorcyclizine	Steroid hormones
Ethchlorvynol	Steroid hormones
Glutethimide	Antipyrine, glutethimide, warfarin
Griseofulvin	Warfarin
Phenobarbital and other barbiturates (secobarbital is an exception)	Barbiturates, chloramphenicol, chlorpromazine, cortisol, coumarin, digitoxin, anticoagulants desmethylimipramine, doxorubicin, estradiol, phenylbutazone, phenytoin, quinine, testosterone
Phenylbutazone	Aminopyrine, cortisol, digoxin
Phenytoin	Cortisol, dexamethasone, digitoxin, theophylline
Rifampin	Coumarin anticoagulants, digitoxin, methadone, glucocorticoids, metoprolol, oral contraceptives, prednisone, propranolol, quinidine

Agents That Inhibit Drug Metabolism in Humans

Inhibitor	Drug whose metabolism is inhibited
Allopurinol, isoniazid Chloramphenicol	Antipyrine, dicumarol, probenecid, tolbutamide
Cimetidine	Chlordiazepoxide, diazepam, warfarin
Dicumarol	Phenytoin
Diethylpentenamide	Diethylpentenamide
Disulfiram	Antipyrine, ethanol, phenytoin, warfarin
Ethanol	Chlordiazepoxide, diazepam, methanol
Grapefruit juice	Alprazolam, atorvastatin, cisapride, Cyclosporine, midazolam, triazolam
Ketoconazole	Cyclosporine, astemizole, terfenadine
Nortriptyline	Antipyrine
Oral contraceptives	Antipyrine
Phenylbutazone	Phenytoin, Tolbutamide
Secobarbital	Secobarbital
Troleandromycin	Theophylline, methylprednisolone

DOSAGE

Abacavir	300 mg bid
Abokinase/Urokinase	A loading dose of 300,000 units orally over 10 minutes & maintenance dose of 300,000 units/hour for 12 hours
Acarbose	25-100 mg before meals
Acebutolol	200-600 mg bid
Acetarsol	500-750 mg bid per vagina for 10 days
Acetaminophen	500-1000 mg qid

Acetazolamide
    Diuretic: 500 mg initially, followed by 250 mg 6 hourly
    Anti-seizure: 10 mg/kg/day, upto 1000 mg/day

Acetylcysteine	200mg sacchet tid
Acetylsalicylic acid	1200-1500 mg, qid
Acitretin: Vit.A derivative	25-50 mg /day
Acriflavine, *Antibacterial, Cream/Lotion*	As required

ACTH
    Diagnostic use:0.25 mg (25 units of porcine ACTH)
    Therapeutic:10-20 units qid (use abandoned)

Activated attapulgite	9-12 g/day
Acyclovir	Oral:400 mg tid or 200 mg 5 times daily
	IV:10-20 mg/Kg 8 hourly
Adalimumab	40 mg evey other week
Adenosine	A bolus dose of 6 mg,then a dose of 12 mg
Adetate calcium disodium	30-50 mg/kg.d, IV infusion for 5 days

Adrenaline
    0.3-0.5 mg (0.3-0.5ml of 1:1000 soln) SC or IM, repeated as required

Albendazole
    Oral:400 mg single dose(repeated for 2-3 days for heavy *ascaris infections* & in 2 weeks for *pinworm* infections)

Alclofenac	1.5-3 g daily
Alcuronium	10-20 mg or more
Aldactazide(Spironolactone 25mg+Hydrochlorothiazide25mg)	Od or qid
Aldactone(Spironolactone 25mg)	1-4 times/day
Alfuzosin	5-25 mg/day

Alpha glucosidase inhibitors

Acarbose	25-100 mg before each meal
Miglitol	25-100 mg before meals

Aloes, powdered	100-300 mg/day
Allopurinol	100 mg/day, later titrated to 300 mg/day
Allantoin: Anti-psoriatic (Alphosyl); Cream/lotion/Shampoo: External use	
Alprazolam	0.25-0.5 mg bid or tid
Almitrine bismesylate	30 mg bid
Alprazolam	0.25-1 mg tid
Alprenolol HCl	100-800 mg/day (oral);IV: 5-20 mg
Alteplase(t-PA)	60 mg in one hour, then 40mg at rate of 20 mg/hour
Altrematine	10 mg/kg/day for 21 days
Aluminium glycinate, Aluminium hydroxide	0.5-1 g repeated as required
Aluminium phosphate	400-800 mg/day
Amantadine	100 mg bid or tid
Amikacin	7.5-15 mg/kg/day
Amiloride HCl	5-10 mg/day

(Lasoride)contains Fsrusemide 40 mg+Amiloride 5 mg;1-2 tab/day
(Moduretic)contains Amiloride 5 mg+Hydrochlorothiazide 50 mg;
Dose:1-4 Tab./day; Syp: 5-20 ml/day

Aminocaproic acid	3-6 g qid
Aminoglutethimide	1 g/day
Aminoglycosides	
Streptomycin	1 g/day, IM
Neomycin	1 g, 6-8 hourly, oral
Kanamycin	1 g, 6-8 hourly, oral
Amikacin	500 mg, IM, 12 hourly
Gentamicin	5-6 mg/kg/d, IV, in three doses or a single dose
Tobramycin	5-6 mg/kg/d, IM or IV, in three doses
Netilmicin	5-7 mg/kg/d, IV, in three doses or a single dose
Aminophylline	Oral: 100-300 mg; PR: 360 mg bid; IV: 250-500 mg/day
Aminosalicylic acid(PAS or para aminosalicylic acid)	8-12 g/day, oral
Amiodarone	100-200 mg/day
Amitriptyline Embonate	50-150 mg/day
Amitriptylene HCl	75-200 mg/day
Amlodipine	5-10 mg, oral, once daily
Ammonium bicarbonate	300-600 mg/day
Ammonium chloride	Upto 6 g/day
Amodiaquine HCl	Suppressive: 400 mg weekly
	Therapeutic: 400-600 mg daily for 3 days
Amoxapine	150-300 mg/day
Amoxycillin trihydrate	750 mg-4.5 g /day

Amphotericin B Systemic fungal disease:0.5-1 mg/kg/day IV infusion
Amphetamine sulphate 5-20 mg/day
Ampicillin 1-8 g/day
Ampicillin trihydrate 1-8 g/day
Ampicillin sodium 1-8 g daily, IM
Amprenavir 1200 mg bid
Amylobarbitone *Hypnotic*: 100-200mg;
Sedative upto 400 mg/day
Amylobarbitone sodium *Hypnotic*: 100-200 mg;
Sedative: upto 600 mg/day
Amyl nitrate, inhalant 0.18-0.3 ml
Androgens & anabolic steroids preparations for replacement therapy
   Methyltestosterone Oral: 25-50 mg/day; SL: 5-10 mg/day
   Fluoxymesterone Oral: 2-10 mg/day
   Testosterone propionate: SL:5-20 mg/d;IM:10-50 mg,3 times/week
   Testosterone enanthate: IM:50 mg every 4,then 3,then every 2 weeks, with each change taking place at 3 months interval.The dose is then doubled to 100 mg every 2 weeks until maturation is complete.Finally adult replacement dose of 200 mg at two weeks interval.
   Testosterone Transdermal: 2.5-10 mg/day
Topical gel(1%): 5-10 g gel/day
Anisotropine 50 mg tid
Anistreplase A single IV inj. of 30 units over 3-5 minutes
Antimony sodium tartrate IV: 500 ml of 0.5% solution
Antimony sodium tartrate IV: Initially 30 mg,increasing by 30 mg on alternate days to a maximum single dose of 120 mg.
Antimony sodium α-α-dimercapto succinate
IM: 30-50 mg/kg BW, maximum of 2.5 g
Anti-TNF-Alpha 5 mg/kg at 0,2 & 6 weeks, repeat every 6-12 weeks
Apazone 600 mg bid
Apomorphine HCl 2-8 mg SC or IM
Aripiprazole 10-30 mg/day
Aromatic ammonia spirit 1-5 ml/day
Ascorbic acid *Prophylactic:* 25-75 mg/day; *Treatment*: 250 mg/day
Aspirin
   Antipyretic/analgesic: 0.3-1 g, upto 4 g/day in divided doses;
   Acute Rheumatism: 4-8 g/day
Atenolol 50-200 mg/day
Atorvastatin 10-80 mg/day
Atracurium 0.3-0.6 mg/kg BW

Atropine	0.4 mg tid or qid
Atropine methobromide, Atropine methonitrate, Atropine sulphate	0.25-2 mg/day, SC, IM, IV, oral
Attapulgite, activated	9-12 g/day
Auranofin (oral gold preparation)	6 mg /day
Aurothioglucose (Parenteral gold preparation)	*Test dose*: 5-25 mg IM; then 50 mg weekly for 20 weeks
Aurothiomalate(Parenteral gold preparation)	Dose same as Aurothioglucose
Azathioprine	(2 mg/kg/day) or100-150 mg/day
Azithromycin	50 mg loading dose,followed by 250 mg a single daily dose for next 4 days.A single 1 g dose is as effective as a 7 days course of Doxycycline for chlamydial cervicitis and urethritis
Bacampicillin	400-800 mg tid
Beclomethasone	4 puffs twice daily (400 mcg/day)
Belladonna herb prepared	30-200 mg/day
Belladonna dry extract	15-60 mg/day
Bendrofluazide	2.5-10 mg/day
Bendroflumethaizide	2.5-10 mg once daily
Benzthiazide	20-100 mg/day in two divided doses
Benzathine penicillin	Prophylactic: 0.9 g every 2 or 3 weeks
Benzhexol HCl	2 mg/day, increased upto 20 mg/day
Benztropine Mesylate	500 mcg/day, increased to 6 mg/day
Benzylpenicillin Sodium/Potassium	0.5-3 g/day, IM
Bephenium Hydroxynaphthoate	2.5 g as a single dose
Bepridil	200-400 mg, oral, once daily
Betamethasone	500-9000 mcg/day
Betamethasone sodium	500-9000 mcg/day
Bethanidine sulphate	10-20 mg/day, increased to 200 mg/day
Betoxolol	10 mg/day
Biperidin	5-20 mg/day by IM or slow IV injection
Bisacodyl	10-15 mg oral; 10 mg suppository; 10 mg/30 ml PR
Bisoprolol	5 mg/day
Bismuth subcarbonate	0.6-2 g/day
Bithionol	30-50 mg/kg/alternate days, 10-15 doses
Bretylium tosylate	5 mg/kg in 10 mnites IV, repeated after 10 minutes
Bromhexine HCl	24-32 mg/day
Bromocriptene	1.25 mg bid, increased upto 7.5-30 mg/day
Brompheniramine	4-8 mg/day
Bumetanide	0.5-2 mg/day
Buprenorphine	0.3-0.6 mg IM, IV 6-8 hourly;0.2-0.4 mg tab SL 6-8 hourly

Bupropion	200-400 mg/day
Buspirone	5-10 mg bid or tid
Busulphan	2-8 mg/day, 150-250 mg course
Butobarbitone	100-200 mg
Butorphanol	1-4 mg/day, IM, IV, SC
Caffeine	100-300 mg/day
Caffeine hydrate	100-300 mg/day
Calcium carbonate	1-2 g/day
Calcium gluconate	1-5 g orally; 1-2 g IM, IV
Calcitonin (Pork)	*Paget's disease*: 40-160 units
	Hypercalcaemia: 640 units, SC or IM
Calcium lactate	1-5 g/day
Calcium sodium lactate	0.3-2 g/day
Capreomycin sulphate	1 g once daily IM, or 15 mg/kg/day
Captopril	25 mg tid initially, increase to 50 mg tid
Carbamezapine	*Anti-seizure*: 15-25 mg/kg (1-2 g per day)
	Antimanic: 200 mg bid, increased as needed
Carbenicillin sodium	12-30 g/day, IV
Carbenoxolone sodium	300 mg daily for one week, then 150 mg/day
Carbimazole	5-45 mg/day in divided doses
Carbidopa 25 mg+Levodopa 100 mg (Sinemet):	upto 25/250 mg tid or qid
Carbinoxamine	4-8 mg/day
Carboplatin	AUC 5-7 mg x min/ml
Carboprost tromethamine	2.5 mg intra-amniotic injection
Carbromal	0.3-1 g/day
Cardamom tincture compound	2-5 ml/day
Carmustine	200 mg/sq.m IV 6 weeks
Carteolol	2.5 mg/day
Carvedilol	6.25 mg bid
Cascara liquid extraxt	2-5 ml/day
Caspofungin	A loading dose of 70 mg, then 50 mg/day, IV
Castor oil	5-20 ml/day
Catechu	0.5-1 g/day
Cefaclor	(10-15 mg/kg/day) 250-500 mg tid
Cefazolin	0.5-2 g tid, IV
Cefditoren pivoxil	200-400 mg bid
Cefepime	0.5-2 g 12 hourly, IV
Cefixime	200 mg bid or 400 mg once daily
Cefoperazone	25-100 mg/kg/day, 8-12 hourly
Cefotaxime	1-2 g 6-12 hourly, IV

Cefotitan	1-2 g bid, IV
Cefoxitin	1-2 g, tid, IV
Cefpodoxime proxetil	200-400 mg bid
Cefrozil	250 mg-1 g /day
Ceftibuten	400 mg once daily
Ceftazidime	1-2 g, 8-12 hourly, IV
Ceftriaxone	1-4 g once daily, IV; (4 g/day for meningitis)
Cefuroxime	0.75-1.5 g tid, IV
Cefuroxime axetil	0.25-0.5 g bid
Celecoxib	100-200 mg bid
Cephadroxil	0.5-1 g bid, oral
Cephalexin, cephradine	0.25-0.5 g qid, oral
Cephaloridine	1-6 g/day, IM
Cephalothin	2-12 g/day
Cephamandole	0.5-2 g, qid
Cephazolin	0.5-1 g, tid
Cephradine	1-4 g/day
Cetrizine	5-10 mg/day
Charcoal, activated	4-8 g/day
Chloral hydrate	0.3-2 g/day
Chlorambucil	6-12 mg daily; maintenance dose 2-4 mg daily
Chloramphenicol	1.5-4 g/day (25-50 mg/Kg BW in children)
Chloramphenicol Palmitate	1.5-4 g/day (25-50 mg/Kg BW in children)
Chloramphenicol sodium	3-4 g daily, SC, IM, IV injection
Chlorcyclizine HCl	50-200 mg daily
Chlordiazepoxide	10-20 mg, bid or tid
Chlorothiazide	0.5-1 g/day in two divided doses
Chlorotrianisene	12-24 mg/day

Chloroquine phosphate
   Suppression of malaria: 500 mg once weekly,
   Treatment of malaria: 600 mg stat followed by 300 mg after 6 hours and 150 mg bid orally, for two days (of base),
   0.5-1 g daily orally and 200-300 mg by IV or IM;
   Rheumatoid arthritis: 0.25-1.5 g daily; Amoebiasis: 0.5-1.2 g daily

Chloroquine sulphate
   Suppression of malaria: 400 mg once weekly;
   Treatment of malaria:0.4-1.2 g daily orally and 200-300 mg, IV or IM;
   Rheumatoid arthritis:0.2-1.2 g/day;*Hepatic amoebiasis*:400-800 mg/day

Chlorpheniramine Maleate   Oral:5-16 mg daily,IM:5-20 mg,single dose

Chlorpromazine   *Psychiatric state*,oral:100-1000mg/day;IM 25-100mg;
   Antiemetic: 25-50 mg oral/IM

Chlorpropamide	100-500 mg daily
Chlortetracycline	1-3 g/day
Chlorthalidone	50-100 mg/day, single dose
Chlorthalidone	100-200 mg daily

Cholecalciferol: *Prophylaxis of Ricklets*: upto 20 mcg daily; *Treatment of Rickets and osteomalacia*:0.125-1.25 mg/day; *Hypoparathyroidism*: 1.25-5 mcg daily:

Choline theophyllinate	400-1.600 mg/day, Maintenance 0.05 ml/minute
Chorionic gonadotrophin	500-5000 units, IM injection
Cimetidine	Oral: 400-800 mg bid;IV:200 mg tid or qid
Ciprofloxacin	500 mg/day or 1500 mg/day in tuberculosis
Cisplatin	20 mg/sq.m/day IV for 5 days or 50-70 mg/sq.m as a single dose every 3 weeks
Citalopram	20-60 mg/day
Clarithromycin	250-500 mg twice daily
Clidinium	2.5 mg tid-qid
Clindamycin HCl	(0.15-0.3 g tid) or 600-1800 mg/day
Clioquinol	0.75-1 g daily
Clofazimine	200 mg/day
Clofibrate	Upto 2 g daily
Clomiphene citrate	50-200 mg/day, starting on 2nd or 3rd day of menstrual cycle, for 5 days
Clomipramine	75-300 mg/day
Clomocycline	170 mg 6 hourly
Clonidine HCl	0.2-1.2 mg/day
Clorazepate, *as a sedative*	5 -7.5 mg bid
Clorazepate dipotassium (*as adjunct to treatment of epilepsy*)	45 mg/day
Cloxacillin sodium	1.5-3 g/day
Clozapine	300-600 mg/day
Codeine, Codeine phosphate	10-60 mg/day
Cod liver oil	Upto10 ml daily
Colchicine	*Prophylactic dose*: 0.6 mg 1-3 times daily *Acute attack*: Start with 0.6-1.2 mg, then 0.6 mg every 2 hours until relief of pain or nausea and diarrhoea appear. **Caution**: By IV route, 8 mg in 24 hours may be fatal.
Colestipol	1-16 g/day
Colesevelam	625 mg upto 6 times/day
Colistin sulphate	Oral: 9-18 mega units daily
Colistin sulphomethate sodium	3-9 mega units daily, IM injection
Corticotrophin injection	40 units once daily
Corticotrophin zinc injection	40 units once daily (250µg-1mg IM)

Cortisol (Hydrocortisone)	20 mg/day
Cortisone Acetate	Oral: 12.5-25 mg daily; Injection: 50-400 mg daily
Cotrimoxazole(400 mg sulphamethoxazole+80 mgTrimethoprim)	2 Tab bid
Cyanocobalamin	1 mg, IM every 3rd day,and then 250 mcg every month
Cyclizine HCl	25-50 mg/day
Cyclobarbitone calcium	200-400 mg
Cyclopenthiazide	250-500 mcg/day
Cyclophosphamide	2 mg/kg/day;(100-150 mg daily)
Cycloserine	0.5-1 g/day in two or three divided doses
Cyclosporine	3-5 mg/kg/day in two divided doses
Cyproheptadine HCl (Periactin)	4-20 mg daily
Dacarbazine	300 mg/sq.m/day IV for 5 days
Danthron	25-50 mg/day
Dapsone	25-300 mg daily
Debrisoquine sulphate	200-300 mg daily
Decamethonium	3-4 mg
Delavirdine	400 mg tid
Demeclocycline	600 mg/day
Desferrioxamine mesylate	IV infusion:15 mg/kg BW per hour, not more than 80 mg/kg in 24 hours; Oral: Gastric lavage with 2 g in 1 litre and leave 10 g in 50 ml fluid in stomach
Desipramine	75-200 mg/day
Deslanoside	IV or IM, initially 0.8-1.2 mg; Maintenance dose 400 mcg every 2-4 hours
Desoxycortisone Acetate	IM injection: 2-5 mg daily Total implantation dose: 100-400 mg
Dexamethazone	0.75 mg orally/day
Dexamethazone sodium phosphate	IM or IV: 4-24 mg
Dexamphetamine sulphate	5-20 mg daily
Dextromethorphan HBr	15-30 mg/day tid or qid
Dextropropoxyphene HCl	Upto 260 mg daily
Dextropropoxyphene Napsylate	Upto 400 mg daily
Diamorphine HCl	5-10 mg/day SC, IM, IV
Diamorphine HCl, tincture	0.25-2 ml/day
Diazepam	*Sedative*: 5-30 mg /day orally, 5-10 mg IM,or slow IV, *Status epilepticus*:IM or slow IV, 10-40 mg & rectally
Diazide(Triamterene50mg+Hydrochlorothiazide25mg)	1 to 4 times/day
Diazoxide	50-150 mg repeated every 5 minutes till blood pressure is lowered;(3 mg/kg BW); 150-1000 mg daily by IV infusion

Dichlorophen	*Adults*: 2-6 g daily for 2 days; *Children*: 2-4 g daily for 2 days
Dichloralphenazone	650-1300 mg as a single dose
Dichlorphenamide	25-50 mg 1 to 4 times daily
Diclofenac	50-75 mg qid
Dicyclomine HCl	10-20 mg qid
Didanosine	250-400 mg qid
Dienoestrol	*Menopausal syndrome*: 50-5000 mcg day; *Cancer*: 15-30 mg daily
Diethyl carbamazine citrate	50 mg (1 mg/kg in children) on day 1, three 50 mg doses on day 2, three 100 mg doses (2 mg/kg in children) on day 3, and then 2 mg/kg tid to complete the 2-3 week course
Diflunisal	500 mg bid
Digitalis prepared	*Rapid digitalisation*: 1-1.5 mg *Maintenance dose*: 50-200 mcg daily
Digitoxin	*Rapid digitalisation*: 0.5-0.75 mg, tid for 3 doses *Maintenance dose*: 0.10 mg daily
Digoxin	*Rapid digitalisation*: Oral: 1-2.5 mg; IV: 0.5-2 mg *Maintenance dose*: Oral: 250-750 mcg; IV: 250 mcg/day
Dihydrocodeine tartrate	30-60 mg/day
Dihydrotachysterol	0.125-1.25 mg daily
Diloxanide furoate	500 mg tid for 10 days or more
Diltiazem	30-80 mg, oral, bid or tid; 75-150 mcg/kg IV
Dimenhydrinate	25-50 mgday
Dimercaprol (B.A.L)	1st day: 400-800 mg IM injection, every 4-6 hours, 200-300 mg on 2nd and 3rd day, and subsequent doses: 100-200 mg
Dinoprostone	*Induction of labor/softening of cervix*: Gel (0.5mg PGE) or controlled-release preparation (10 mg PGE2); *Abortifacient*: 20 mg vaginal suppository, repeated 3-5 hours
Diphenhydramine HCl	50-300 mg daily
Diphenoxylate	*Lomotil* (2.5 mg Diphenoxylate+Atropine 0.025 mg) 2 Tab 6 hourly
Disopyramide	150 mg tid or 1 g/day
Disopyramide phosphate	Oral: 300 mg loading dose, then 100-150 mg 6 hourly IV injection: 100-150 mg, then 25 mg/hour by infusion to a maximum of 500 mg daily
Disulfiram	800 mg/day, then decrease slowly over 5 days

	to 100-200 mg daily for upto a year
Dopamine	2-20 mcg/Kg BW per minute, IV infusion
Dothiepin HCl	75-50 mg daily
Doxazocin	1-4 mg once daily
Doxiphin HCl	75-300 mg/day
Doxycycline	First dose 200 mg, then 100 mg once daily
Doxylamine	1.25-25 mg/day
Dronabinol	5 mg/square meter
Droperidol	5-20 mg/day
D-Tubocuraine	30 mg IV
Dyrenium (Triamterene 50mg)	1-3 times daily
Efavirenz	600 mg qid
Emetine HCl	30-60 mg/day
Edrophonium Chloride	IV injection 2 mg followed by 8 mg
Emetine HCl	30-60 mg daily, SC or IM injection
Enalapril	5 mg, then 10-20 mg daily
Enfuvirtide	90 mg bid SC
Enoxacin	400 mg/day
Ephedrine/Ephedrine HCl	15-60 mg/day orally
Epinephrine	0.4ml of 1:1000 solution SC or inhaled 320 mcg/puff
Epoetin alfa, Erythropoietin (Epogen, Procrit)	50-150 IU/kg/day
Eplerenone	50-100 mg/day
Ergocalciferol	*Prevention of Rickets*: Maximum 20 mcg daily(800 units)
	Treatment of rickets and osteomalacia:0.25-1.25 mg daily
Ergometrine Maleate	Orally: 0.5-1 mg/day
	IM: 0.3-1 mg;IV:0.1-0.5 mg/day
Ergotamine tartarate	Oral: 1-2 mg;SC or IM : 0.25-0.5 mg
Ertapenem	1 g/day, IM or IV
Erythromycin	1-4 g/day
Eryhtromycin Estolate	1-4 g daily
Eryhtromycin Stearate	1-4 g daily
Erythropoietin	50-300 IU/kg three times a week IV, SC
Escitalopram	10-30 mg/day
Esmolol	Loading dose:0.5-1 mg/kg,then constant infusion first 50-150 mcg/kg/min, increased every 5 min upto 300 mcg/kg/min
Esomeprazole	20-40 mg/day

Estrogens
    Ethinyl estradiol   0.005-0.02 mg/day
    Micronized estradiol   1-2 mg/day
    Estradiol cypionate   2-5 mg every other week
    Estradiol valerate   2-30 mg every other week
    Estropipate   1.15-2.5 mg/day
    Conjugated, esterified, or mixed estrogenic substances
        Oral   0.3-1.25 mg/day
        Injectable   0.2-2 mg/day
        Transdermal, Patch
    Diethylstilbestrol   0.1-0.2 mg/week
    Quinestrol   0.1-0.2 mg/week
    Chlorotrienestril   12-25 mg/day
    Methallenestril   3-9 mg/day
Estrogen inhibitors and antagonist: Tamoxifen   10-20 mg bid
Etanercept   25 mg twice weekly
Ethacrynic acid   50-200 mg daily
Ethambutol   15-25 mg/kg/day; 50 mg/kg twice a week
Ethinyloestradiol   *Menopause*: 10-50 mcg daily;
         Cancre: 100-1000 mcg daily
Ethionamide   0.5-1 g daily or 15 mg/kg/d
Ethisterone   25-50 mg daily
Ethosuximide   750 mg daily, increasing to 2 g/day
Ethylmorphine HCl   6-30 mg/day
Ethyloestrenol   2-4 mg daily
Etidronate   7.5 mg/kg in saline infusion/day for 3 days
Etodolac   200-300 mg qid
Ezetimibe   10 mg once daily
Famciclovir   Oral: 250 mg bid or tid
Famotidine   20 mg bid
Fazadinium   0.75-1 mg/kg BW
Felbamate   2000-4000 mg/day
Felodipine   5-10 mg, oral, once daily
Fenfluramine HCl   40-120 mg/day
Fenofibrate   54 mg tablet once daily or tid
Fenoldopam   0.1-1.6 mcg/kg/min by IV infusion
Fenoprofen   600 mg qid
Fentanyl citrate   10-60 mcg, IV
Ferrous fumarate   *Prophylactic*: 200 mg daily;
         Therapeutic: 400-600 mg daily

Ferrous gluconate	*Prophylactic*: 600 mg daily
	Therapeutic: 1.2-1.8 g daily
Ferrous succinate	*Prophylactic*: 200 mg daily
	Therapeutic: 400-600 mg daily
Ferrous sulphate	*Prophylactic*: 300 mg daily
	Therapeutic: 600-900 mg daily
Ferrous sulphate, dried	*Prophylactic*:200 mg daily
	Therapeutic: 400-600 mg daily
Fexofenadine (Allegra)	60 mg/day
Flecainide	100-200 mg bid
Flucloaxacillin sulphate	1-2 g daily
Fluconazole	100-800 mg/day
Flucytosine	100-200 mg/kg/day
Fludrocortisone acetate	1-2 mg initially, maintenance:100-200 mcg daily or 0.1 mg 2-7 times weekly (has potent salt retaining activity)
Flufenamic acid	600 mg daily
Fluoroquinolones	
Nalidixic acid	250-500 mg bid
Ciprofloxacin	500 mg, divided in two doses
Clinafloxacin	200 mg
Enoxacin	400 mg
Levofloxacin	500 mg
Gatifloxacin	400 mg
Lomifloxacin	400 mg
Moxifloxacin	400 mg
Norfloxacin	400 mg, divided in two doses
Ofloxacin	400 mg, divided in two doses
Travofloxacin	200 mg
Fluprednisolone	1.5 mg/day
Fluoxetine	10-60 mg/day
Fluoxymesterone	1-2 mg daily
Fluphenazine decanoate	12.5-60.5 mg, IM at intervals of 14-35 days
Fluphenazine enanthate	12.5-25 mg, IM at intervals of 10-28 days
Fluphenazine HCl	*Anxiety states*: 1-2 mg daily
	Schizophrenia: 2-60 mg daily
Fluprednisolone	2 mg/day
Flurbiprofen	300 mg tid
Fluticasone	Inhale upto 2000 mcg/day
Fluvastatin	20-40 mg once daily
Fluvoxamine	100-300 mg/day

Folic acid	*Prophylactic*: 200-500 mcg daily (during pregnancy)
	Therapeutic: 1 mg/day (in megaloblastic anaemia)
Fomivirsen	*Induction*: 330 mcg every 2 weeks, then every 4 weeks
Foscarnet	40 mg/Kg 8-12 hourly, IV
Fosfomycin	Single 3 g dose
Furazolidone	400 mg daily
Furosemide	Oral: 20-80 mg/day;IV: 20-40 mg/day
Gabapentin	2400 mg/day(*Post-herpetic neuralgia*:1800 mg and above)
Gallamine triethiodide	80-120 mg or more as required
Gallium nitrate	200 mg/sq.meter body surface area/day,IV infusion
Ganciclovir	IV: 5 mg/kg twice or five times daily
	Oral: 1 g tid;Inraocular implant:4.5 mg every 6-8 months
Gatifloxacin	400 mg/day
Gemfibrozil	600 mg once or twice daily
Gentamicin sulphate	80-240 mg/day IM injection
Ginger tincture	0.25-5 ml/day
Ginger tincture, weal	1.5-3 ml/day
Glibenclamide (Gliburide)	2.5-20 mg once daily
Glimeperide	0.001-0.004 g/day
Glipizide (Glydiazinamide)	0.005-0.04 g/day
Glucagon	SC, IM, IV injection: 0.5-1 Unit
Glutethimide	250-500 mg/day
Glyceryl trinitrate	0.5-1mg sublingual stat, maximum 6 mg/day
Glycopyrrolate	1 mg bid-tid
Gold	See aurothiomalate & aurothioglucose
Gonadorelin	SC, IM, IV injection: 100-500 units
Griseofulvin	500-1000 mg/day, with fatty foods
Growth hormone (Somatotropin)	1 mg(3 units) once daily in evening
Guanethidine monosulphate	10-20 mg/day,increasing to 25-50 mg daily
Halazepam (Paxipam)	20-40 mg, bid or qid
Haloperidol	Oral: 2-60 mg/day
Halquinol	1.5-2 g daily
Heparin calcium	*Prophylactic*: SC, 10,000-15000 units daily
Heparin sodium	*Prophylactic*: SC, 10,000-15000 units/day
	Treatment:IV, 20,000-60,000 units daily
Hexamethomine	5-25 mg SC or IV
Hyaluronidase	
	IV 500-1000 units with each 500-1000 ml of infusion fluid;
	Local anaesthesia: 1000 units for 20ml of anaesthetic solution
Hydralazine	40-200 mg/day

Hydrochlorothiazide	25-50 mg/day
Hydrocodone	5-10 mg/day
Hydrocortisone	20 mg/day
Hydrocortisone acetate:	Intra-articular injection or local infiltration 5-50mg
Hydrocortisone sodium phosphate	100-500 mg IV injection
Hydrocortisone sodium succinate	100-500 mg IV injection
Hydroflumethiozide	25-50 mg daily
Hydroxychloroquine sulphate	
Suppression of malaria:	400 mg once weekly
Treatment of malaria:	0.4-1.2 g daily
Rheumatoid arthritis:	0.2-1.2 g daily (6.4 mg/kg/day)
Hydrochlorothiazide	25-100 mg/day, single dose
Hydroflumethaiazide	25-100 mg/day, in two divided doses
Hydroxycobalamin	Initially 1 mg, repeated 5 times at intervals of 2 or 3 days; Maintenance dose: 1 mg every 2 months
Hydroxyprogesterone hexamoate	250-500 mg, IM injection, once or twice weekly
Hydroxyurea	20-30 mg/Kg
Hydroxyzine	15-100 mg/day
Hyoscine butylbromide	30-100 mg/day
Hyoscine hydrobromide	300-600 mcg/day
Hyoscine methobromide	5-15 mg daily
Ibuprofen	1200-1600mg/day & upto 2400 mg/day
Imipenem	0.25-0.5 g 6-8 hourly, IV
Imipramine HCl	75-200 mg/day
Indapamide	2.5-10 mg/day, as single dose
Indinavir	800 mg tid
Indomethacin	75-100 mg/day; 100 mg PR
Infliximab	3-10 mg/kg after every 8 weeks
Inspra (Elerenone25.50mg)	1-2 times daily
Insulin	According to the need of the patient
Iodide, orally	150-200 mcg/day
Iodoquinol	650 mg tid for 21 days
Ipanoic acid	2-6 g as a single dose before radiographic examination
Ipecacuanha tincture	0.25-1 ml; Prepared: 25-100 mg
Ipratropium	1-2 puffs (18-36 mcg)
Isoniazid	Oral: 300-600 mg/day; IM: 100-300 mg/day or 5-10 mg/kg/day *Tubercular meningitis*: Upto 1 g twice weekly

Isoprenaline sulphate	5-20 mg sublingualy or by inhalation in solution
Isopropamide	5 mg bid
Isoproterenol	Inhaled 80-120 mcg
Isosorbide dinitrate, sublingual (SL)	0.5-6 mg/day
Isosorbide dinitrate, sublingual, long acting	2.5-10 mg/2 hours
Isosorbide dinitrate, oral	10-60 mg per 4-6 hours
Isosorbide dinitrate, chewable oral	5-10 mg per 2-4 hours
Isosorbide mononitrate, oral	20 mg per 12 hours
Isoxuprine HCl	*Vasodilator*: 80 mg daily
	Premature labour: IV infusion 0.2-0.5 mg/minute for 12 hours followed by 10 mg IM every 3 hours
Ispaghula Husk	3-5 g bid or tid
Isradipine	2.5-10 mg oral, every 12 hours
Itraconazole	100-400 mg/day
Ivermectin	150 mcg/kg, single dose, every 6-12 months
Kanamycin acid sulphate	0.5-1mega unit/day, IM injection
Kaolin, light	15-75 g/day
Ketoconazole	200-1200 mg/day
Ketoprofen	70 mg tid
Ketorolac	10 mg qid
Ketotifen	1 mg bid
Labetalol	Oral: 200-2400 mg/day;
	Hypertensive emergencies: 20-80 mg,repeated IV bolus
Lamivudine	150-300 mg bid or qid
Lamotrigene	100-300 mg/day
Lanatoside C	Initial dose for *rapid digitalisation*: 1000-1500 mcg
	Maintenance dose: 250-750 mcg/day
Lansoprazole	30 mg/day
Levallorphan Tartrate	*Mother*:04-08 mg, IV as a single dose
	Neonate: 10 µg/kg BW, IV
Levamisole HCl	175 mg as a single dose
Levodopa:Initially 250 mg/day,increased to maintenance dose 2.5-8 g/day	
Levodopa 100 mg+ Carbidopa 25 mg (Sinemet), upto 250/25 mg tid or qid	
Levofloxacin	500-750 mg/day, in one or two doses daily
Levorphanol tartrate	Oral: 1.5-4 mg; SC or IM: 2-4 mg; IV:1-1.5 mg
Levopropoxyphene napsylate	Oral: 50-100 mg bid or tid
Levothyroxine	*Hypothyroidism*: 1-6 months age:10-15 mcg/kg/day
	Adults: 1.7 mcg/kg/day
	Myxedema coma:300-400 mcg IV,then 50 mcg/day
Lidocaine	Infusion:150-200 mg in 15 minutes,then 2-4 mg/minute

Lignocaine HCl	50-100 mg, maintained by 1-2 ml/minute, IV
Lincomycin HCl	Oral: 1.5 g daily, 30 minutes before food
	IM inj: 0.6-1.2 g daily in 2 doses
	IV infusion: 600 mg every 8 hours
Linezolid	600 mg twice daily, oral or IV
Liothyronine sodium	37.5 mcg daily
Liquid paraffin	10-30 ml once daily
Lisinopril	10-80 mg/day
Lithium carbonate	0.5 mEq/kg/day in divided doses
Lomifloxacin	400 mg/day
Lomustine	150 mg/sq.m orally every 6 weeks
Lopinavir+Ritonavir	(400 mg+100mg) bid
Loracarbef	(10-15 mg/kg/day) 250-500 mg tid
Loratadine	10 mg/day
Lorazepam	1-2 mg once or bid
Losartan	25-100 mg/day
Lovastatin	10-80 mg/day
Loxapine	20-160 mg/day
Lugol's iodine	Oral: 150-200 mcg/day
Lymecycline	Oral: 204 mg bid
Magnesium carbonate/oxide	*Antacid*: 250-500 mg; *Laxative*: 2-5 g
Magnesium sulphate	*Antacid*: 5-15 g
Magnesium trisilicate	0.5-2 g repeated as required
Magnesium as sulphate (in cardiac arrhythmias)	1 g IV in 20 mniutes

Mannitol
    12.5-25 g every 1-2 hours to maintain urine flow rate greater than 100 ml/hour (upto 50 g/day slow IV infusion)

Maprotiline	75-300 mg/day
Maxzide(Triamterene 75mg+Hydrochlorothiazide 50mg)	Once daily
Maxzide-25mg(Triamterene27.5mg+Hydrochlorothiazide25mg)	Once daily

Mebendazole
    Pinworms: 100 mg once, repeated at 2 weeks
    Ascariasis, trichuriasis, hookworm: 100 mg, bid for 3 days
    Intestinal capillariasis: 400 mg/day for 21 or more days

Mechlorethamine	0.4 mg/kg IV in single or divided doses
Meclizine HCl (Bonine)	25-50 mg/day
Meclofenamate	100 mg qid
Medioxyprogesterone heavy	Oral: 2.5-4 mg daily
	IM: 50-150 mg; *Neoplasms*: 100-400 mg daily

Mefenamic acid	1.5 g daily
Mefloquine	*Prophylactic for malaria*: 250 mg weekly
Meloxicam	7.5-15 mg qid
Melphalan	Oral: 2-15 mg daily; IM: upto 100 mg single dose
Mepacrine HCl	*Suppression of malaria*: 100 mg daily
	Treatment of malaria: 200-500 mg daily
	Tapeworm: 1 g in divided doses
	Giardiasis: 300 mg daily for 5 days
Mepenzolate	25-50 mg qid
Meperidine	80-100 mg/day
Meprednisone	4 mg/day
Meprobamate	400-1200 mg daily
Mepyramine maleate	Oral: 300-600 mg daily
	IM, IV inj: 25-50 mg
Mercaptopurine	100-200 mg daily
Meropenem	1-2 g 8 hourly (2 g 8 hourly for meningitis),IV
Mersalyl	(sodium salt of mersalyl acid+theophylline) IM: 0.5-2ml
Metaraminol tartrate	SC or IM: 2-10 m;IV inj: 2.5-5 mg
	IV infusion:upto 100 mg dissolved in 500 ml of normal saline or dextrose infusion
Metformin HCl	500 mg-2.55 g day
Methacycline	600 mg/day
Methadone HCl	5-10 mg orally or IM/day
Methallenoestril	*Menopause*: 9 mg daily; *Cancer*: 3-18 mg daily
Methamdienon	5-10 mg daily
Methantheline	50-100 mg qid
Methaqualone	75 mg tid or qid
Methazolamide	50 mg 1-4 times daily
Methicillin	1 g tid or qid, IM, IV
Methimazole	30 mg, once daily,maintenance dose:5-15 mg once daily
Methisazone	6 g daily
Methoserpidine	Initial dose: upto 30 mg daily
	Maintenance dose: upto 60 mg daily
Methotrexate	IM, IV: 15-25 mg weekly
	Intrathecally: 5-10 mg
Methoxamine HCl	IM: 5-20 mg; IV inj.:5-10 mg
Methscopalamine	2.5 mg qid
Methyclothiazide	2.5-10 mg/day as a single dose
Methyldopa	Oral: 1-2 g/day
Methyldopate HCl	IV: 250-500 mg

Methylphenobarbitone	Upto 350 mg daily
Methylprednisolone	(0.5mg/kg every 6 hours); 4-48 mg daily
Methylprednisolone acetate	4 mg/day
Methyltestosterone	25-50 mg daily for a *man*
	5-20 mg daily for a *woman*
	Mammary carcinoma: 50-100 mg daily
Methyprylone	200-400 mg daily
Methysergide maleate	1-2 mg bid or tid
Metoclopramide HCl	10-20 mg qid orally or IV
Metoprolol	100-400 mg/day
Metformin	0.5-2 g/day in divided doses
Metolazone	2.5-10 mg/day as a single dose
Metrifonate	7.5-10 mg/kg tid at 14 days interval
Metronidazole	750 mg tid, or 500 mg IV, 6 hourly for 10 days
Mesoridazine	50-400 mg/day
Metyrapone	300-500 mg every 4 hours, total of six doses
Mexiletine	600-1200 mg/day
Midamor(Amiloride 5mg)	Once daily
Miglitol	25-100 mg before meals
Migril	1 tab qid
Minocycline	100 mg once or bid
Minoxidil	*As antihypertensive*: 40 mg/day
Mirtazapine	15-60 mg/day
Mitotane	12 g/day
Moduretic(Amiloride5mg+Hydrochlorothiazide50mg)	Once or twice daily
Molindone	20-200 mg/day
Moricizine	200-300 mg, oral, tid
Morphine sulphate/Morphine Hcl	10-20 mg orally, SC or IM
Moxifloxacin	400 mg/day
Mustine HCl	400 mcg/Kg Inj. into the fast running saline IV infusion
Mycophenolate mofetil (MMF)	Upto 2 g/day
Nabumetone	1000-2000 mg once daily
Nadolol	40 mg/day
Nalbuphine	10 mg/day
Nalidixic acid	2-4 g /day in divided doses
Nalorphine Hydrobromide	IV inj: 5-10 mg (total dose: 40 mg)
Naloxone HCl	0.4 mg IV repeated at 2-3 minutes interval as required
Nandrolone decanoate	IM: 50-50 mg
Nandrolone phenylpropionate	IM: 25-50 mg weekly
Naproxen	250-1000 mg daily

Nateglinide	60-120 mg before meals
Nefazodone	200-600 mg/day
Nelfinavir	750 mg tid or 1250 mg bid
Neomycin sulphate	1.4-4.2 mega units daily
Neostigmine bromide	15-30 mg tid or as needed by patient
Neostigmine methyl sulphate	0.25-2 mg SC or IM/day
Netilmicin	5-7 mg/kg/day
Nevirapine	200 mg bid
Niacin	See Nicotinic Acid
Nicardipine	20-40 mg, orally, 8 hourly
Niclosamide	2 g once, chewed and swallowed
Nicotinamide	Prophylactic: 15-30 mg daily
	Therapeutic: 50-250 mg daily; IV inj. 50-250 mg
Nicotinic, acid	*Heterozygous familial hypercholestrolemia*: 2-6 g/day
	Hypercholestrolemia & hypertriglyceridemia: 1.5-3.5 g/day
	Prophylactic: 15-30 mg daily
	Therapeutic: 50-250 mg daily
Nicoumalone	Initial dose: 12-20 mg, subsequent dose 2-12 mg in accordance with the prothrombin activity of the blood
Nifedipine	20-40 mg, oral, 8 hourly; 30-90 mg/day; 3-10 mcg/kg/IV
Nikethamide	0.5-2 g, IV
Nimodipine	60 mg, oral, every 4 hours
Nisoldipine	20-40 mg, oral, once daily
Nitrazepam	5-10 mg/day
Nitrendipine	20 mg, oral, once or twice daily
Nitrofurantoin	400 mg daily
Nitroglycerin, sublingual	0.15-1.2 mg
Nitroglycerin, oral sustained action	6.5-13 mg per 6-8 hours
Nitroglycerin 2% ointment, transdermal	1-1.5 inches per 4 hours
Nitroglycerin, slow-release, buccal	1-2 mg per 4 hours
Nizatidine	150 mg bid
Nor-adrenaline acid tartrate: 8-12 mcg/min, IV infusion, repeated as required	
Norethisterone	5-20 mg daily
Norethisterone acetate	2.5-20 mg daily
Norfloxacin	400 mg/day
Northendrolone	20-50 mg daily
Nortriptyline HCl	75-150 mg daily
Noscapine	15-30 mg tid or qid
Nutmeg oil	0.05-0.2 ml
Nystatin	*Alimentary moniliasis*: 1-2 mega units daily

Octreotide	50 mcg/hour, IV
Oestradiol benzoate	1-5 mg daily, IM Inj.
Ofloxacin	400 mg/day
Olanzapine	10-30 mg/day
Omeprazole	20 mg/day
Opium, Tincture	0.25-2 ml;(Opium, powdered: 25-200 mg)
Orciprenaline sulphate	Oral: 20-80 mg daily; SC, IM: 500 mcg
Orphenadrine citrate/HCl	200-400 mg daily
Ouabain (a glycoside of strophanthus)	0.12-0.25 mg IV
Oxamniquine	15 mg/kg bid for 2 days
Oxaprozen	1200-1800 mg/day as single dose
Oxazepam	15-30 mg tid or qid
Oxazolidinediones: Linezolid	600 mg twice daily
Oxprenolol HCl	160-480 mg/day in divided doses
Oxybutynin	5 mg tid
Oxycodone	4.5 mg/day
Oxymetholone	Oral:5-30 mg daily,*Aplastic anaemia*: 100-350 mg daily
Oxymorphone	1-1.5 mg, repeated as required
Oxyphenbutazone	200-400 mg daily
Oxyphencyclimine	10 mg bid
Oxyphenonium	5-10 mg qid
Oxytetracycline dihydrate	1-3 g/day
Oxytetracycline HCl	Oral: 1-3 g daily;IV infusion: 1-2 g daily
Pamidronate	60-90 mg infusion in 2-4 hours
Penciclovir	Topical: Apply 2 hourly
Pancreatin	2-8 g daily with meals
Pancuronium bromide	4-6 mg or more
Pantoprazole	40 mg/day
Paracetamol	0.5-1 g/day
Paraffin liquid	10-30ml
Para-aminosalicylic acid(PAS)	(300 mg/kg BW);10-20 g daily
Paraldehyde	Oral: 5-10 ml; IM Inj: 5-10 ml;PR: 15-30 ml,diluted
Paramethasone	2 mg/day
Paromomycin	*Intestinal amebiasis*: 10 mg/kg tid for 7 days
Paroxetine	20-50 mg/day
Penbutolol	20 mg/day
Penicillamine	Oral: 150 mg once a week
Penicillins	
Penicillin G	1-4 mega units 4-6 hourly,IV
Penicillin VK	0.25-0.5 g qid,oral

Cloxacillin	0.25-0.5 g qid,oral
Nafcillin	1-2 g 4-6 hourly,IV
Oxacillin	1-2 g 4-6 hourly,IV
Amoxicillin	0.25-0.5 g tid,oral
Amoxicillin/pot.clavulanate	500/125,875/125 bid,tid,oral
Piperacillin	3-4 g,4-6 hourly,IV
Ticracillin	3 g,4-6 hourly,IV
Pentamidine isethionate	Prophylactic: IM inj:300 mg every 3-6 months
	Therapeutic: 150-300 mg daily for 7-15 days
Pentazocine	30-60 mg/day
Pentazocine HCl	25-100 mg after food
Pentobarbitone	100-200 mg
Pentobarbitone sodium	100-200 mg
Pentolinium tartrate:	SC:1 mg first dose,then according to requirement
Peppermint oil	0.05-0.2 ml/day
Pergolide	0.05 mg/day, increased to 3 mg/day
Perphenazine	*Antipsychotic*: 8-64 mg daily
	Antiemetic: 4 mg tid; IM: 5-10 mg
Pethidine HCl	Oral: 50-100 mg;SC or IM:25-100 mg;IV: 25-50 mg
Phenazone	300-600 mg/day
Phenelzine sulphate	45-75 mg/day
Phenethicillin potassium	0.5-1.5 g daily
Phenformin HCl	50-200 mg daily
Phenindamine tartrate	75-150 mg daily
Pheniramine maleate	75-150 mg/day
Phenobarbital(Luminal sodium)	15-30 mg bid or tid
Phenobarbitone	Upto 350 mg/day in divided doses
Phenobarbitone sodium	Oral: Upto 350 mg daily;IM or SC inj: 50-200 mg
Phenolphthalein	50-300 mg/day
Phenoxymethyl Penicillin	0.5-1.5 g daily
Phentolamine mesylate	IV : 5-10 mg
Phenylbutazone	Oral: 200-400 mg daily
	PR: 250 mg once or twice daily
Phenylephrine HCl	IV:0.8 mg;IM,SC:5 mg;Oral:250mg
Phenylpropanolamine HCl	75-150 mg daily
Phenytoin sodium	Oral: 300 mg/day,increasing (each time 25-30 mg)
	to 400 mg daily according to needs of the patient.
	IM or slow IV(Fosphenytoin): Upto 250 mg
Pholcodine	30-60 mg/day
Phosphate	50 mmol or 1.5 g over 6-8 hours
Phthalasulphathalazole	5-10 g daily

Physostigmine	1-2 mg
Phytomanadione	*Antidote to oral anticoagulants*: 5-20 mg
	Haemorrhagic disease of newborn:IM,IV:0.5-1 mg
Pilocarpine	SC, Oral:3-12 mg
Pioglitazone	15-45 mg once daily
Pindolol	10-40 mg/day
Piperazine adipate/citrate/phosphate	
	Adults: *Threadworms*: 1-2 g, once daily for 2 days
	Roundworms: 4.5 g, single dose
	Children: *Threadworms*: 40 mg/Kg
	Roundworms: 120 mg/Kg, as single dose
Piperazine hydrate:	*Adults*: 2 g daily
	Children: Upto 6 years 250 mg for each year of age
	6-12 years: 1.5 g daily
Piperacillin	100-150 mg/kg/day in two doses
Pirenzepine	50 mg bid
Piroxicam	20 mg/day, a single dose
Pivampicillin	0.5-1 g bid
Poldine methylsulphate	1-30 mg daily
Polymyxin B sulphate	500,000 units 8 hourly, IM
Polythiazide	1-4 mg daily, as a single dose
Potassium bromide	1-6 g daily
Potassium chloride	Oral: 50 mEq/day; IV: 10-30 mEq/hour
Potassium iodide	
	Expectorant: 250-500 mg
	Preoperative treatment of thyrotoxicosis: 150 mg/day
	Non-toxic goitre: 10 drops, orally/day
Pralidoxime chloride	1-12 g/day
Pramipexole	0.125 mg tid, increased upto 0.5-1.5 mg tid
Pravastatin	Upto 80 mg/day
Prazepam	10-20 mg bid or tid
Praziquantel	10-20 mg/Kg for 2-3 doses with intrval of 4-6 hours
Prazocin	10-30 mg/day
Prednisolone	5-60 mg/day
Prednisolone pivalate	*Intraarticular injection or local infiltration*: 5-20 mg
Prednisolone sodium/phosphate	IV: 20-100 mg once or bid
Prednisone	*Bronchial asthma*:30-60 mg/day,oral;1 mg/kg/6 hourly IV
Prenylamine lactate	180-300 mg daily
Primaquine phosphate	15 mg/day for 14 days
Primidone	10-20 mg/kg/d or(0.5 g daily, increasing to 1-2 g/day

Probenecid	Start with 0.5 g orally/day in divided doses and increased to 1 g/day after one week
Procainamide HCl	IV loading dose:12 mg/kg at the rate of 0.3 mg/kg/min, then 2-5 mg/min (2-5 g/day)
Procaine Penicillin	300-900 mg/ day, IM
Procarbazine	50-200 mg/day orally
Prochlorperazine maleate	*Antipsychotic*: 15-100 mg daily *Antiemetic*:15-25 mg
Prochlorperazine mesylate	*Antipsychotic*: 12.5-25 mg BD or TDS,IM inj *Antiemetic*: 12.5 mg,IM inj.
Procyclidine HCl	7.5 mg daily increasing to 30 mg
Progesterone	IM: 20-60 mg daily
Progesterone inhibitor and antagonist	
	Mifepristone: 400-600 mg/day for 4 days or 800mg/day for 2 days
	Danazol:600 mg/day,then decreased to 400 mg and later 200 mg/day
Proguanil HCl	As suppressant of malaria:100-300 mg daily
Promazine HCl	20-50 mg daily
Promethazine HCl	10-25 mg/day
Propafenone	450-900 mg in three doses
Propantheline	15 mg qid
Propiverine	15 mg bid or tid
Propoxyphene	60-120 mg/day
Propranolol HCl	80-480 mg/day oral; 3-10 mg slow IV
Propylthiouracil	100-150 mg 6-8 hourly
Protriptyline	20-40 mg/day
Pyrantel pamoate	11 mg/Kg(maximum,1 g) single dose,repeat after 2 week
Pyrazinamide	20-30 mg/kg/day; 50-70 mg/kg twice a week
Pyridoxine HCl	100-300 mg/day
Pyrilamine	25-50 mg/day
Pyrimethamine	25-50 mg/week
Quetiapine	150-800 mg/day
Quinine HCl /Quinine sulphate	
	Prophylaxis of malaria: 300-600 mg daily
	Treatment of malaria: 1.2-2 g daily;IV Inj: 300-600 mg
Quinine	Oral dose of quinine & its salts: 325 mg qid for 7 days; *For babesia species(protozoal infection)*:650 mg for 7 days *Prophylaxis of P.falciparum*: 600 mg daily from the day prior to exposure to at least a month after departure from an endemic area

P.falciparum coma: Initial IV dose of 20 mg/kg BW given over 4 hours, then 10 mg/kg BW as a 4-hours infusion every 8 hours

Quinine sulphate	Oral dose of quinine & its salts: 325 mg qid for 7 days
Quinethazone	50-100 mg/day as a single dose
Quinupristin-dalfopristin	7.5 mg/kg every 8-12 hours, IV
Rabeprazole	20 mg/day
Radioactive iodine	80-120 µCi/g of estimated thyroid weight corrected for uptake
Ranitidine	150 mg bid
Refocoxib	12.5-50 mg as a single dose
Repaglinide	0.25-4 mg/day, maximum 16 mg/day before meals
Reserpine	*Antihypertensive*: 100-500 mcg (0.1-0.5 mg) daily
	Antipsychotic: 1-5 mg daily
Resuvastatin	10-40 mg/day
Reteplase	IV bolus injection of 10 units; another bolus after 30 minutes
Rhubarb powder	0.2-1 g/day
Rhubarb tincture compound	5-15 ml/day
Riboflavine	*Prophylactic*: 1-4 mg daily
	Therapeutic: 5-10 mg daily
Riboflavine sodium phosphate	*Prophylactic*: 1-4 mg daily
	Therapeutic: 5-10 mg daily
Rifabutin	300 mg/day
Rifampin/Rifampicin	600 mg/day single dose
Rifapentine	600 mg once or twice weekly
Risperidone	4-16 mg/day
Ritonavir	600 mg bid
Ropinirole	0.25 mg tid, increased upto 2-8 mg tid
Rosiglitazone	2-8 mg once daily
Salbutamol	*Bronchodilator*:
	Oral: 6-10 mg daily
	IV infusion: 3-20 mcg/ml
	Slow IV: 350 mcg
	Premature labour: IV infusion: 10-45 mcg/ml
Salcatonin	*Paget's disease*: SC or IM: 50-100 units
	Hypercalcaemia: SC or IM: Upto 400 units
Saquinavir hard gel	600 mg tid

Saquinavir hard gel	1200 mg tid or 1800 mg bid
Scopalamine	0.4 mg tid
Selegiline	5 mg with breakfast and 5 mg with lunch
Senega infusion	Oral: 2.5-5 ml
Senega liquid extract	0.5-2 ml
Senega fruit powdered	0.5-2 g
Senega leaf powdered	0.5-2 g
Sermorelin (*Synthetic human growth hormone*)	0.03 mg/kg once daily
Sertraline	5-200 mg/day
Serum gonadotrophin	IM inj according to the requirement
Simvastatin	5-80 mg/day
Sodium aminosalicylate	10-15 g daily
Sodium aurothiomalate	IM: 10-50 mg/week, total 1 g
Sodium bicarbonate	Antacid: 1-5 g/day
Sodium calcium edetate	Upto 4 g daily
Sodium citrate	Upto 10 g daily
Sodium cromoglycate	Oral: 20 mg qid & by inhalation
Sodium fusidate	1-2 g daily
Sodium iodide/iodate	
	Expectorant: 250-500 mg/day
	Preoperative treatment of thyrotoxicosis:150 mg/day
	Nontoxic goitre:1 g orally per day
Sodium nitroprusside	0.5-10 mcg/kg/min;20-200 mcg/ml,IV infusion
Sodium salicylate	5-10 g/day (Acute rheumatism)
Sodium stibogluconate	0.6-2 g daily for 10-30 days,IM,IV
Sodium sulphate	5-15 g/day
Sodium thiosulphate	25 g, IV
Sodium valproate	200-800 mg tid
Somatostatin	250 mcg/hour,IV
Sorbitol	IV : Upto 6 g/ml
Sotalol	200-600 mg/day
Spearmint oil	0.05-2 ml
Spectinomycin	40 mg/kg,single dose(upto a maximum of 1 g)
Spironolactone	100-400 mg daily
Squill, liquid extract	0.06-0.2 ml
Squill powdered	60-200 mg
Squill elixir	2.5-5 ml
Stanolone	50-75 mg daily
Stavudine	30-40 mg bid

Stilboestrol	*Menopausal symptoms*: 100-1000 mcg daily
	Cancer treatment: 3-20 mg daily
Streptogramins(Quinupristin+dalfopristin)	7.5 mg/kg every 8-12 hours, IV
Streptokinase	Loading dose: 150,000 units IV infusion, then 100,000 units/hour for 24 to 72 hours
Streptomycin sulphate	0.5-1 G/day, (15 mg/kg/day), IM or IV
Succinylsulphathiazole	10-20 g daily
Sucralfate	1 g four times daily, 1 hour before meals
Sufentanil	0.02 mg
Sulfamethoxazole	1 g 2 or 3 times daily
Sulfinpyrazone	200 mg orally/day; later 400-800 mg/day
Sulfisoxazole	1 g 4 times daily
Sulindac	200 mg bid
Sulphadiazine	Oral: 1 g qid; IM or IV: 4 g daily
Sulphadoxine	1 g, single dose
Sulphadoxine+Pyrimethamine	3 Tablets, single dose
Sulphadimethoxine:	Initial dose: 1-2 g, Subsequent dose: 500 mg daily
Sulphadimidine	2-6 g daily
Sulphadimidine sodium	1-2 g, IM or IV
Sulphafurazole	*Systemic infections*: 3-6 g daily
	Urinary tract infections: 2-4 g daily
Sulphamethizole	100-200 mg 4 or 6 hourly
Sulphamethoxydiazine	Initial dose: 1-2 g, later 500 mg daily
Sulphamethoxypyridazine	Initial dose: 1 g, later 500 mg daily
Sulphapyridine	0.5-3 g/day
Sulphasalazine	2-3 g/day
Sulphathiazole	2-6 g daily
Sulphinpyrazone	200-600 mg daily
Sulphabromophthalein sodium	IV: 2-5 mg/Kg
Sulphopnylureas	
Tolbutamide	0.5-2 g in divided doses
Tolazamide	0.1-1 g single or divided doses
Chlorpropamide	0.1-0.5 g single dose
Gliburide(Glibenclamide)	0.00125-0.02 g/day
Glipizide	0.005-0.04 g/day
Glimepiride	0.001-0.004 g/day
Sulthiane	Upto 600 mg daily

Suxamethonium Bromide	According to requirement of patient
Suxamethonium Chloride	According to requirement of patient
Talampicillin	250-500 mg 8 hourly
Telithromycin	800 mg once daily
Tenecteplase	A single IV bolus of 0.5 mg/kg
Tenofovir	3 00mg qid
Terazocin	5-20 mg/day
Terbinafine	250 mg/day
Terbutaline	Oral: 1.5-5 mcg/day;0.25 mg IV
Testosterone	Total implantation dose: 100-600 mg
Testosterone phenylpropionate	IM : 5-25 mg once or twice daily
Testosterone propionate	IM : 5-25 mg once or twice daily
Tetrachlorethylene	*Hookworm*: 1-2 ml as asingle dose
Tetracosactrin acetate	250 mcg, IM
Tetracycline HCl	Oral: 1-3 g/day;IV:0.1-0.5 g 6-12 hourly
Thiabendazole	1.5 g, twice daily for 2-3 days
Thianbutosine	500 mg daily, increasing every 14 days by 500 mg to a maximum of 2 g daily
Thiamine HCl	*Prophylactic*: 2-5 mg daily
	Therapeutic: 25-100 mg daily
Thiazolidinediones	
Pioglitazone	15-45 mg once daily
Rosiglitazon	2-8 mg once daily
Thioamides	See Methimazole & Propylthiouracil
Thiopentone sodium	IV: 100-500 mg/Kg
	Per rectum: 40 mg/Kg, maximum dose 2 g
Thioridazine HCl	100-800 mg daily
Thiothixene	2-120 mg/day
Thiotepa	IV injection: 15-30 mg, repeated as required
Thymoxamine HCl	160-480 mg daily
Thyroxine sodium	150-200 mcg/day
Tigabine	16-56 mg/day
Timolol maleate	30 mg/day
Tincture aurantie (orange)	1-2 ml/day
Tincture belladonna	0.5-2 ml/day
Tincture camphor co	2-10 ml/day
Tincture camphorated opium, concentrated	0.25-1.25 ml/day
Tincture cardamom co	2-5 ml/day

Ticture chloroform and morphine	0.3-0.6 ml/day
Tincture ginger strong	0.25-0.5 ml/day
Tincture ginger weak	1.5-3 ml/day
Tincture hyoscyamus	2-5 ml/day
Tincture ipecacuanha	0.25-1 ml/day
Tincture nux vomica	0.5-2 ml/day
Tincture opium	0.25-2 ml/day
Tincture rheubarb compound	Upto 15 ml daily in divided doses
Tincture squill	0.3-2 ml/day
Tincture stramonium	Upto 6 ml daily in divided doses
Tinidazole	1-2 g daily
Tobramycin	210-350 mg/day, IM, IV or 5-6 mg/kg/day
Tolazamide	100-500 mg/day
Tolazoline HCl	Upto 200 mg daily
Tolbutamide	0.5-2 g daily
Tolmetin	400 mg qid
Tolterodine	2 mg bid
Topiramate	Start with 50 mg/day, increase to 200-600 mg/day
Torsemide	2.5-20 mg/day
Tranylcypromine sulphate	20 mg/day, increased upto 60 mg/day
Trazodone	50-600 mg/day
Triamcinolone	4 mg/day
Triamterene	150-250 mg/day
Triclofos sodium	0.5-2 g as a single dose
Trichlormethiazide	2-8 mg/day, as a single dose
Tridihexethyl	25-50 mg tid or qid
Trifluperazine HCl	*Antipsychotic*: 5-60 mg; *Antiemetic*: 1-6 mg daily
Trifluridine	Topical:1 drop every 2 hours or apply 5 times daily
Trimeprazine tartrate	1-50 mg/day
Trimetaphen	3-4 mg/min. IV
Trimethadione	30 mg/kg/day
Trimethobenzamide	250 mg orally;200 mg rectally;200 mg IM
Trimethoprim	100 mg bid or 100-300 mg/day single dose
(Trimethoprim 160mg+Sulphamethoxazole 800mg)	1 tablet bid
Trimipramine maleate	75-200 mg daily
Tripelennamine(PBZ)	25-50 mg/day
Triprolidine HCl	5-7.5 mg/day
Trovafloxacin	200 mg/day

Troxidone	*Adults*: 900-1800 mg daily; *Children*: 300-900 mg daily
Tubocurarine chloride	30 mg or according to need of the patient
Unithiol	3-5 mg/kg, IV every 4-6 hours
Valacyclovir	Oral: 500 mg-1 g bid or tid
Valdecoxib	10 mg as a single dose
Valganciclovir	900 mg bid or tid
Valproic acid & sodium valproate	*Antiepileptic*: 30-60 mg/kg/day *Antimanic*: Start with 750 mg/day, increased to 1500-2000 mg
Vancomycin HCl	500 mg 6 hourly, IV infusuion
Venlafaxine	75-225 mg/day
Verapamil	240-480 mg/day; 75-150 mcg/kg IV
Vigabatrin	500 mg bid, a total of 2-3 g/day
Vinblastine sulphate	10 mg, IV weekly
Vincristine sulphate	*Adults*: 25-75 mcg/Kg/Week *Children*: 30-150 mcg/Kg weekly
Viprynium embonate	5 mg/Kg as a single dose
Vitamin D	4000 units/day
Voriconazole	400 mg/day, oral
Warfarin sodium	Start with 5-10 mg daily, later 5-7 mg/day
Wild cherry syrup	2.5-10 ml/day
Zafirlukast	Oral: 10 mg once daily
Zalcitabine	0.75 mg tid
Zidovudine	200 mg tid or 300 mg bid
Zileuton	Oral: 600 mg qid
Ziprasidone	80-160 mg/day
Zolidronate	4 mg infused in 15 minutes
Zonisamide	100-600 mg/day (4-12 mg/day in children)

INDEX

Acne Preparations	131
Active Immunisation agents availabe in USA	107
Acute Methanol or Ethylene Glycol Poisoning	46
Adrenal Steroid Inhibitors	20
Adrenoceptor-activating and other Sympathomimetic Drugs	13
Adrenocortical Antagonists	74
Adrenocorticosteroids	73
Alcohol Abuse, Drugs for Prevention	46
Acute Alcohol Withdrawal Syndrome	46
Alpha (α) Blockers	17
Anaemias; Haematopoietic Growth Factors	63
Anaesthetics:	
General Anaesthetics	47
Local Anaesthetics	49
Analgesics	
Narcotic Analgesics	59
Non-narcotic Analgesics (NSAIDs)	68
Analgesic Combinations	59
Common Opioid Analgesics	60
Androgens & Anabolic Steroids	76
Angiotensin Convertuing Enzyme Inhibitors	22
Angiotensin Receptor Blockers	23
Anthelmintic Drugs (Antihelminthics)	95-98
hookworm, roundworm (ascaricides), threadworms, tapeworm (taenicides), filariasis, schistosomiasis	
Anti-Alzeheimer Drugs	53
Anti-Amoebic Drugs (amoebicides)	92
Anti-Anginal Drugs	29
Anti-Anxiety drugs (Minor Tranquillizers)	55
Anti-Arrhythmic Drugs (Cardiac arrhythmias)	31
Antibiotics	81
Anti-Cancer Drugs	99-103
Anticholinergic Drugs	11

Anticholinesterases	10
Anti-Coagulants	65
Anti-Depressants	56
Anti-Diabetic Drugs	77
Anti-Diarrheal Drugs	111
Anti-Emetics & Emetics	113,114
Anti-Epileptic Drugs/Anti-sizure Drugs	46
Anti-Fungal Agents (Systemic & Topical)	94
Anti-Histamine, Serotonin & Ergot alkaloids	37
Anti-Hypertensive Drugs	21
Anti-Inflammatory Agents	68
Anti-Inflammatory (selected drugs) for GIT Diseases	119
Anti-Inflammatory Agents (Dermatological)	132
Anti-Leprosy Drugs	109
Anti-Lipidemic Drugs	67
Anti-Malarials (treatment and prophylaxis)	91
Anti-Neoplastic	99-103,132
Anti-Platelet Drugs (Anti-Thrombotic Drugs)	66
Anti-Protozoal Drugs	91
amoebicides (antiamoebic drugs)	92
anti-malarials (treatment and prophylaxis)	91
giardiasis (anti-giardial drugs)	93
leishmaniasis (leishmanicides)	93
trichomoniasis (trichomonacides)	93
Anti-Pruritic Agents	132
Anti-Psychotics/Major Tranqullizers/Neuroleptics	54
Anti-Rheumatic Drugs (disease modifyning anti-rheumatics)	69
Anti-Schizophrenic Drugs	54
Anti-Seborrhoea Agents	111
Anti-Tussives	97
Anti-Viral Agents (Systemic & Topical)	86
classification according to mechanism of action	
therapeutic classification	
Appetite Suppressants	113
Autonomic Drugs	9
Benzodiazepines	55
Beta (β) Blockers(selectivity, solubility, duration of action)	19

Bitters	115
Blood, Inflammation, Gout	63
Bone Mineral Homeostasis	80
Bronchial Asthma	40
Bronchodilators	42
Calcium Channel Blockers	22
Cancer Chemotherapy/Anti-Cancer Drugs	99-103
Carbonic Anhydrase Inhibitors	116
Cardiac Arrhythmias	31
Cardiovascular-Renal Diseases	21
Central Nervous System	44
Central Nervous System Depressants	60
Central Nervous System Stimulants	13
Chemotherapeutic Drugs	81
Cholinergic Drugs (Parasympathomimetics)	9
Cholinestrerase Inhibitors (therapeutic uses/duration of action)	11
Cholinergic Blocking Drugs (Antimuscarinic or Cholinoceptor Blocking)	12
Colitis & Crohn's Disease	112
Congestive Cardiac Failure See Heart Failure	30
Dermatologic Pharmacology	130
Digestants	111
Digestive Enzymes	111
Disaese-Modifying Anti-Rheumatic Drugs (DMARDs)	69
Diseases of blood, Inflammation, and Gout	63
Disinfectants, Antiseptics and Sterilants	89
Diuretics	33
Dosage Schedule	134-162
Drugs acting on smooth muscle (Antihistamines, Serotonin, & Ergot Alkaloids)	37
Drugs of Abuse	61
Drugs that act in the Central Nervous System	44
Drugs during Lactation and their Effects on the Nursing Infant	128
Ecto-Parasiticides	131
Eicosanoids (Prostaglandins, Thromboxanes, Leukotrienes,etc.)	39
Emetics	114

Endocrine Drugs	71
Erectile Dysfunction	129
Ergot Alkaloids	39
Estrogens	75
Expectorants/Mucolytics	116
Filariasis	96
Fibrinolytics (Thrombolytic Drugs)	66
Gall Bladder, Gallstones Dissolving Agents	117
Gastrointestinal Tract, drugs acting on	119
General Anaesthetics	47
Giardiasis (Antigiardial Drugs)	93
Glaucoma (open angle)	98
Glucocorticoids	75
Goitre, Nontoxic	73
Gonadal Hormones/Antagonists & Inhibitor	76
Gout	69
Haemostatics (Coagulants)	64
Heart Failure	30
Heavy Metal Intoxication & Chelators	108
H1-Receptor Antagonists	37
Hookworm	95
H. Pylori Disease	120
Hyperlipidemia (Anti-lipidemics)	67
Hyperthyroidism (Antithyroid Agents)	72
Hypothalamic & Anterior/Posterior Pituitary Hormones	71
Hypothyroidism (Thyroid Agents)	71
Immunoglobulins	110
Immunopharmacology	105
Immunomodulants/ Immunomodulators 106	
Agents for Active Immunisation availabe in USA	107
Infantile Spasms	47
Inflammatory Bowel Disease(Crohn's disease,Ulcerative colitis)	112
Inhibitors of Angiotensin	23
Insulins	77
Iron Preparations, oral	63
Irritable Bowel Syndrome (IBS)	112

Keratolytic and Destructive Agents	132
Kinins (Vasodiltor Polypeptides)	39
Lactation, drugs used during,and their effects on nursing infant	128
Laxatives/Purgatives	123
Leishmaniasis (Leishmanicides)	93
Leprosy, Antileprosy Drugs	109
Local Anaesthetics	49
Malaria in travellers, drugs for prevention	92
Mood Stabilizers	58
Motility Disorders & Selected Anti-Emetics	123
Narcotic Analgesics	59
Neuroleptics	54
Non-Steroidal Anti-inflammatory Drugs (NSAIDs)	68
Nontoxic Goitre	73
Obesity	130
Open angle Glaucoma	118
Opioid Analgesics	60
Organic Nitrites & Nitrates	30
Osteoporosis	129
Pancreatic Hormones and Antidiabetic Drugs	77
Parasympatholytic Drugs	12
Parkinsonism & other Movement disorders	52
Peptic ulcer / H.pylori	119,120
Peptic Ulcer (Acid-Peptic Disease)	120
Peri-natal and Paediatric Pharmacology	126
Pigmentation	131
Poisons and their Antidotes	108
Posterior Pituitary Hormones	71
Progestins	75
Pruritis	132
Psychiatric Disorders	53
Psoriasis	131
Psychotropic Drugs	53
antipsychotics (Major Tranquillizers)	54
anti-anxiety drugs (Minor Tranquillizers)	55
anti-depressants	56
Psychomimetic (Hallucinogens, Psychodelic Drugs)	51

Purgatives	123
Renal Drugs (Diuretics)	33
Respiratory Stimulants (Analeptics)	117
Rheumatic Diseaese (Disease Modifyning Anti-Rheumatics)	59
Roundworm (Ascaricides)	96
Schistosomiasis	96
Schizophrenia	54
Seborrhoea	132
Sedative-Hypnotics; dosage for Sedation and Hypnosis	44,45
Sialogogues/Anti-Sialogogues	122,123
Skeletal Muscle Relaxants	50
Smooth Muscle, drugs acting on:(Antihistamines, Serotonin, & Ergot Alkaloids)	37
H1-Receptor Antagonists, Ergot Alkaloids	
Kinins (vasodiltor Polypeptides), Substance P(undecapeptide)	
Eicosanoids (Prostaglandins,Thromboxanes,Leukotrienes)	
Substance P (undecapeptide)	39
Sunscreens	131
Sympathomimetics	13
according to receptors, according to mode of action, chemical classification and therapeutic classification	
Tapeworm (Taenicides)	96
Threadworms	96
Thyroid storm (Thyrotoxic crisis)	72
Toxicology (See Heavy Metals & Poisoning)	108
Tranquillizers	54,55
Trichogenic & Anti-Trichogenic Agents	132
Trichomoniasis (Trichomonacides)	93
Tuberculosis	104
Vaccines and Sera (Immunological Products)	110
Varices Hemorrhage	110
Vasodilators & Treatment of Angina Pectoris	24,29
Vasoconstrictors	27
Venereal Diseases	109
Viral Diseases	86